Tooth Extraction

Tooth Extraction
A Practical Guide

Paul D. Robinson BDS MB BS FDS RCS PhD
Senior lecturer/consultant
Department of Oral and Maxillofacial Surgery
Guy's, King's and St Thomas' School of Dentistry
London, UK

With a Foreword by **David Poswillo**
Emeritus Professor of Oral and Maxillofacial
Surgery, University of London, UK

wright

OXFORD   AUCKLAND   BOSTON   JOHANNESBURG   MELBOURNE   NEW DELHI

WRIGHT

ELSEVIER

An imprint of Elsevier Limited

© 2000, Elsevier Limited. All rights reserved.

First published 2000
Reprinted 2002, 2005, 2006, 2007

ISBN 13: 978-0-7236-1071-7
ISBN 10: 0-0-7236-1071-1

British Library Cataloguing in Publication Data
A catalogue record for this book is available from the British Library

Library of Congress Cataloging in Publication Data
A catalog record for this book is available from the Library of Congress

Notice

Knowledge and best practice in this field are constantly changing. As new research and experience broaden our knowledge, changes in practice, treatment and drug therapy may become necessary or appropriate. Readers are advised to check the most current information provided (i) on procedures featured or (ii) by the manufacturer of each product to be administered, to verify the recommended dose or formula, the method and duration of administration, and contraindications. It is the responsibility of the practitioner, relying on their own experience and knowledge of the patient, to make diagnoses, to determine dosages and the best treatment for each individual patient, and to take all appropriate safety precautions. To the fullest extent of the law, neither the Publisher nor the Editors/Authors assumes any liability for any injury and/or damage to persons or property arising out or related to any use of the material contained in this book. It is the responsibility of the treating practitioner, relying on independent expertise and knowledge of the patient, to determine the best treatment and method of application for the patient.

The Publisher

your source for books, journals and multimedia in the health sciences

www.elsevierhealth.com

Working together to grow libraries in developing countries

www.elsevier.com | www.bookaid.org | www.sabre.org

ELSEVIER   BOOK AID International   Sabre Foundation

Transferred to Digital Printing in 2010

Contents

Acknowledgements

I would like to thank Paul Sheppard and Simon Nocton for their advice and help in preparation of the manuscript, Andrew Dyer for taking the photographs, Mark de Pienne for the diagrammatic artwork and Eric Whaites for the loan of some of the radiographs.

PDR

Foreword

In the 30 years that have elapsed since the publication of the second edition of Howe's *The Extraction of Teeth* there have been many changes in the practice of dentistry. Prevention has been practised to an increasing extent and many teeth have been restored with a considerable number of new materials. The population has grown older and fewer teeth have been extracted per person than previously. But the fundamental principles of dental extraction remain and the clinical dental student must learn these before placing forceps on a tooth, an opportunity which arises much less frequently today than it did in 1970! Many students graduate with very little experience of extraction under local or general anaesthesia, and intravenous sedation was seldom practised until the 1980s and 1990s. There is, therefore, a need for an updated version of this basic text and it would be hard to fault this edition which covers in a crisp, concise and easily read manner all that the dental surgeon, be it a student or a younger practitioner, must know if the procedure is to be done in a careful and uncomplicated way. Nothing of importance is omitted and the techniques described are illustrated with superb diagrams and photographs. This short text is easy to read and all the tips and traps of exodontia are plain to see.

It will be of immense benefit to the dental student and all practitioners who have the need to extract teeth under local anaesthesia, oral or intravenous sedation and general anaesthesia. No practitioner, however much he feels that he is an expert exodontist, can fail to learn from this edition which is concise but full of wisdom. It does not expand into the more sophisticated areas of surgical dentistry and does not need to do so, for there are plenty of large new tomes and colour atlases that cover these subjects

I recommend the book to all who wish to learn all there is to know about the extraction of teeth in the young and the elderly, and I do so without hesitation or reservation. It is not just a book to read in your dental library – it is a book for everyday use! Buy it and be grateful that in the moment of need – and that shall surely come to all who extract teeth – you have the answer to all the problems you are likely to encounter!

David Poswillo
CBE DSc DDS MDhc FDS FFD FRCPath
Emeritus Professor of Oral and Maxillofacial Surgery
University of London

Preface

This practical manual of tooth extraction aims to be an approachable and easily digestible instruction book, principally for the undergraduate dental student. Based on Geoffrey Howe's original text written in the 1970s, this book contains many of the timeless fundamentals of exodontia so well described by Professor Howe nearly 30 years ago, and read by generations of students since then. But in addition to retaining the unchanged principles underpinning the extraction of teeth, the techniques of surgical management described take note of the changes that have taken place in many areas of practice such as the use of general anaesthesia, and the changing medico-legal climate.

The accent throughout the book is on explanation of practical methods, overcoming mechanical obstacles during surgery, and ways of avoiding problems. With this goal in mind, the text is liberally illustrated with photographs and diagrams to assist the reader in understanding topics from assessment of operative difficulty and patient management, via choice of instruments and technicalities of surgical technique, to the last post-operative complication.

As well as the conventional and the orthodox, there are some thoughts and techniques included that could be described as tricks of the trade; ideas and concepts that have crystallized out of teaching received and experience gained by the author, whose hope is that students of dental surgery at all levels will find something of value within these pages.

Paul D. Robinson

Chapter 1
Introduction

Tooth extraction remains an essential component of both the art and science of dentistry despite the enormous progress in the prevention of dental disease made during the last three decades of the twentieth century. The effects of the fluoride revolution and increasing public awareness of oral health, mean that people in the western world are keeping their teeth longer and fewer teeth are being extracted, particularly in adolescents and young adults. This trend towards the retention of the natural dentition into later life is resulting in more extractions being needed in older patients who have more complicated medical histories and tougher, more brittle bone than the young. Thus the difficulty and complexity of extraction procedures is increasing with the average age of our patients.

Dental surgeons, especially those in training, are required to face these challenges in an exacting medico-legal climate in which litigation looms large when complications arise for whatever reason. It is therefore more important than ever that the principles and techniques of removing teeth are understood by all those in the dental profession who would pick up a pair of extraction forceps.

Having a tooth extracted may also pose a daunting challenge to patients whose imagination of what is to happen could get the better of them. A calm, reassuring approach by the dental surgeon whilst explaining the procedure goes a long way towards allaying such fears and building their confidence. The successful outcome of tooth extraction depends not only on the surgeon's practical skills, but also on his or her ability to empathize with patients and the way they perceive the problem.

INDICATIONS FOR TOOTH EXTRACTION

Teeth may need to be removed for a variety of reasons: the tooth itself is diseased, the tooth is involved in disease affecting surrounding tissues, or the tooth is in the wrong place. Below are some examples:

- Caries may render a tooth unrestorable.
- Pulpitis.
- Periodontal disease.
- Periapical infection/dental abscess.
- Fracture of the tooth.
- Failure of a large restoration.
- Endodontic failure.
- Dental erosion, attrition or abrasion.
- Abnormalities of tooth development, e.g. hypoplasia gemination.
- Root resorption.
- Orthodontic reasons – normally space creation for alignment of other teeth.
- Prosthetic considerations – to facilitate provision of fixed or removable prostheses.
- Impacted or ectopic teeth.
- Teeth involved with cysts or tumours of the jaws.
- Teeth in the direct field for radiotherapy to the jaws may be removed prophylactically.
- Teeth in the line of a jaw fracture may require removal.

METHODS OF TOOTH EXTRACTION

There are two basic methods of tooth removal. The first, which is suitable for the majority of erupted teeth, is extraction using dental forceps. This technique relies on the ability to gain sufficient grip on the root of the tooth by forcing the blades of the instrument into the periodontal space between the root and the alveolar bone. Access to the periodontal space may be facilitated by the use of dental elevators before the forceps are applied. Using this method, the route of approach to the root is solely from inside the tooth socket within the alveolar bone, and hence the alternative name of 'intra-alveolar extraction' (see Chapter 2).

The second method is reserved for those teeth whose roots either cannot be approached and gripped using the forceps technique, or when the roots defy all efforts to deliver them from the bone despite sound application of the forceps. In these cases, bone must be removed from around the roots by dissection through the alveolus after the overlying soft tissues have been reflected as a mucoperiosteal flap. This approach is therefore 'trans-alveolar' (see Chapter 3), but is more commonly called 'the surgical method'.

MECHANICAL PRINCIPLES OF EXTRACTION

1. Applying displacing force to a tooth or root

(a) Direct application using dental forceps, the blades of which grip the root to be removed (Figure 1.1).
(b) Indirectly via a fulcrum (also called a 'point of application') on the bone adjacent to the root using elevators (Figure 1.2).

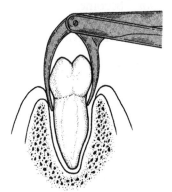

Figure 1.1. Forceps blades engaging and grasping the root to provide a direct displacing force on the tooth.

2. Expansion of the socket using lateral displacing movements that gently widen the socket by distortion of the bone.

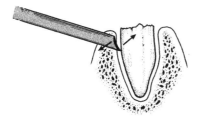

Figure 1.2. Elevator applying displacing force to a root and an equal and opposite force to the fulcrum on adjacent bone.

This action can be likened to removing a post set in the ground. If the soil is loose then the post hole is easily made wider by displacement of its walls. If the ground however is densely compacted, the attempts to shift the post sideways may be resisted completely, and increasing the force applied may at best have no effect and at worst may break the post! Similarly the texture of bone surrounding teeth varies in its compliance and elasticity, this being maximal in the young and tending to decrease with age. Unfortunately the teeth themselves may also become more brittle in older patients, and the combination of these factors has lead to the mirthful but accurate comparison of removing such teeth in mature patients with extracting 'glass from concrete'.

3. Removal of bone surrounding the root   becomes necessary if the socket cannot be expanded sufficiently to permit delivery of the tooth. The options for bone removal involve the use of:

(a) Dental burs (suitably cooled with irrigant spray).
(b) Chisels used with gentle hand pressure or in conjunction with a mallet (for use under general anaesthesia only).

4. Sectioning the tooth   into its component parts; either separating roots one from another or dividing the crown from the root mass may allow removal of the individual components separately whereas the intact tooth may defy any attempts to move it.

PRE-OPERATIVE ASSESSMENT

Time spent assessing the problem pre-operatively is never wasted, hence the old saying in carpentry 'measure twice, cut once'. The assessment should encompass the following aspects of both the surgical task and the patient.

The surgery

The crown of the tooth

- Present/absent/fractured/carious – this may affect the ability to apply forceps to the root as the plane of the periodontal space is less well defined and more difficult to access with the forceps (Figure 1.3).
- Restorations – particularly if these are large and may weaken the tooth.
- Attrition of the crown often indicates a brittle tooth (with a calcified pulp) set in dense bone.
- Accessibility of the tooth in the mouth.

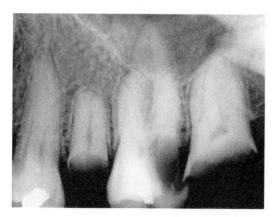

Figure 1.3. Carious crown of upper first molar and absent crowns from two adjacent teeth, each making forceps placement difficult.

(a)

(b)

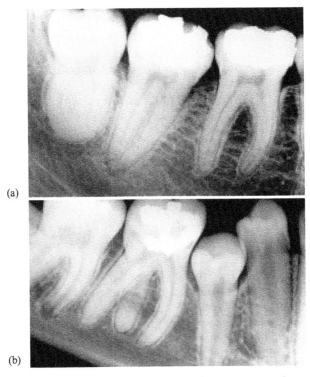

Figure 1.4. (a) Three lower molar teeth with varying root patterns that would offer different degrees of resistance to displacement. (b) Three abnormally curved and splayed roots of a lower first molar.

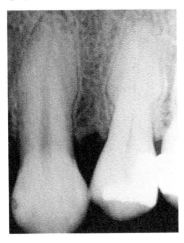

Figure 1.5. Roots of upper canine and first premolar showing hypercementosis.

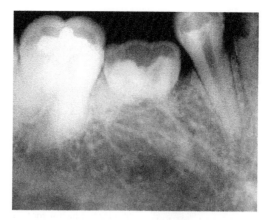

Figure 1.6. Residual roots of lower deciduous molar ankylosed to surrounding bone – the tooth has submerged as a result.

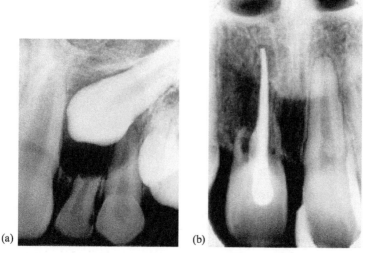

(a)   (b)

Figure 1.7. (a) Physiological resorption of deciduous teeth, facilitating their removal. (b) Pathological resorption of this incisor root leaving a potentially brittle remnant of root.

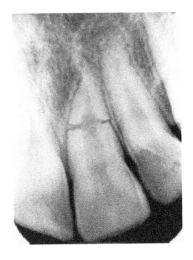

Figure 1.8. Fracture through mid third of a central incisor root – retrieval of the apical portion will require a trans-alveolar approach.

The root of the tooth

- Size – length/width.
- Number of roots.
- Shape of individual roots as well as the collective root mass (Figure 1.4a, b).
- Mobility as assessed clinically.
- Hypercementosis (Figure 1.5).
- Ankylosis (Figure 1.6).
- Resorption (Figure 1.7a, b).
- Fracture of root (Figure 1.8).
- Vitality of the pulp/presence of a root filling or post restoration.

Surrounding bone

- Bone level around the root (Figure 1.9a, b).
- Texture of bone as judged by the radiodensity (opacity), and how closely packed the trabeculae appear on the radiograph (Figure 1.10a, b).
- Loss of bone due to discrete pathological lesions or generalized osteoporosis/atrophy: potential risk of jaw fracture (Figure 1.11).

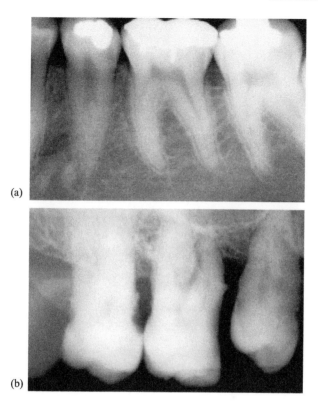

(a)

(b)

Figure 1.9. (a) Alveolar bone crest at the level of the amelo–cemental junction of teeth in the posterior mandible. (b) Bone level near the apical third of roots of teeth in the posterior maxilla.

Nearby structures

- Position of nerves – inferior alveolar, mental (Figure 1.12a, b).
- Maxillary antrum (Figure 1.13).

Radiographs

Many of the points listed above can only be assessed on a radiograph. It is not essential to take a pre-operative X-ray view of every tooth to be extracted, but a radiograph is highly

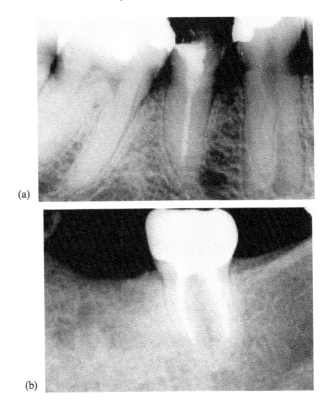

(a)

(b)

Figure 1.10. (a) Bone with a sparse 'open weave' trabecular pattern.
(b) Bone showing a tightly packed dense trabecular pattern.

desirable in the following circumstances:

- History of difficult or failed extractions.
- Any tooth abnormally resistant to removal with forceps.
- When the tooth is to be removed by the trans-alveolar (surgical) method, either as an elective decision pre-operatively or when failure of forceps extraction dictates this.
- Teeth in potentially close proximity to the maxillary antrum/inferior alveolar or mental nerve.
- All mandibular third molars. The roots of these teeth are often abnormal in shape or size and may be related to the inferior alveolar bundle (Figure 1.14a).

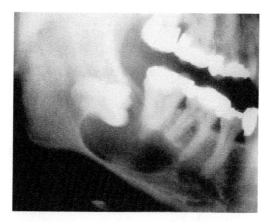

Figure 1.11. Large dentigerous cyst associated with an impacted lower third molar. The mandible is weakened in the molar region by the presence of the cyst.

- All impacted, buried or misplaced teeth (Figure 1.14b).
- Heavily restored or non-vital teeth – the roots may be very brittle (Figure 1.15).
- When any local or generalized bone disease is suspected.
- Teeth that have been subjected to trauma – the root or alveolar bone could be fractured.
- Lone-standing maxillary molars. The bone around their roots may be sclerotic and brittle and the antral cavity is often large in the older patient, so predisposing to fracture of the alveolus creating a communication from the socket into the nasal sinus (Figure 1.16).
- When abnormalities of tooth development may be present (Figure 1.17).
- Patients who have received radiotherapy to the jaws and are therefore at risk of osteoradionecrosis.

Assessment of the patient

Level of co-operation

Most patients will consent to a dental extraction under local anaesthesia following appropriate explanation of what is

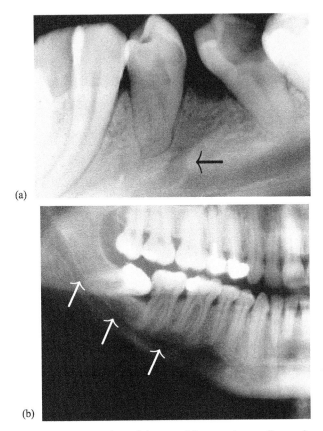

(a)

(b)

Figure 1.12. (a) Shadow of the mental foramen (arrowed) seen close to the root apex of a lower premolar. (b) Inferior dental canal (arrowed) in close proximity to roots of lower molars, particularly the third molar.

planned, and will be adequately co-operative so that the procedure can be undertaken safely and within a reasonable amount of time. When this is in doubt for any reason, consideration should be given to using intravenous sedation, inhalational sedation, or general anaesthesia. In the case of young children below the age of reason, some handicapped patients and those with irreconcilable dental phobia, a general anaesthetic may be the only option. Sedation as an adjunct to local anaesthesia is an effective half-way house for the people who would make good patients but for their

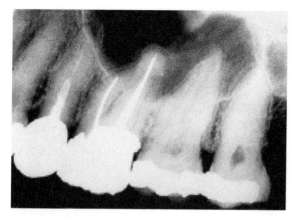

Figure 1.13. Roots of upper cheek teeth (second premolar to third molar) closely related to the maxillary antrum.

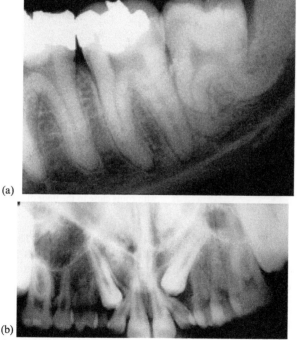

(a)

(b)

Figure 1.14. (a) Erupted lower third molar with three curved roots – potentially an unpleasant surprise for the unwary exodontist without a pre-operative radiograph. (b) Impacted upper canines – the radiograph gives vital information about the position, depth, angulation and relations of these teeth.

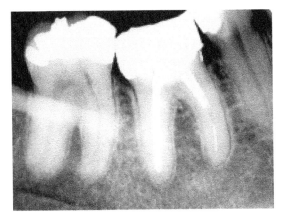

Figure 1.15. Heavily restored, root-filled lower molar set in dense bone.

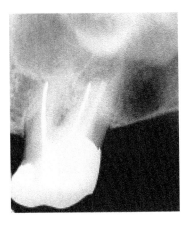

Figure 1.16. Lone-standing upper molar with roots close to the floor of the antrum.

anxiety. Failure to assess the patient adequately in this regard may turn a relatively simple extraction into a complicated problem of management and even lead to an inability to complete the procedure.

Medical history

A thorough medical history must be taken from all patients for dental extraction, both to ensure that it is safe to embark on the surgery and to choose the appropriate type of

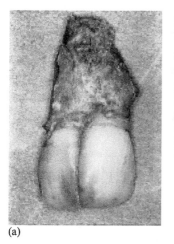

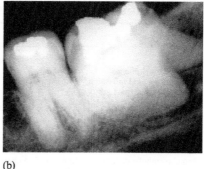

(b)

(a)

Figure 1.17. (a) Gemination of two upper incisors. (b) Gemination of lower second and third molars – forming a tooth mass that would resist extraction until after the removal of a great deal of surrounding bone or sectioning of the tooth mass. (c) A collection of potential surprises! Buried teeth fused to roots of extracted upper molars.

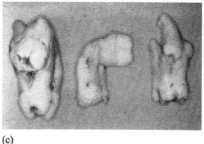

(c)

anaesthesia. Table 1.1 gives some important examples of the types of medical condition giving rise to potential problems with dental extractions, and the necessary avoiding action to be taken.

From Table 1.1 it can be seen that the contraindications to extractions performed under local anaesthesia are very few, and most of these can be managed in hospital by suitable specialists. Notably these include:

1. Bleeding problems – clotting defects (e.g. haemophilia), low platelet counts, patients on anticoagulants.
2. Immunocompromised patients who are susceptible to infection – leukaemias, patients having chemotherapy for malignant disease, late stage AIDS (acquired immuno-deficiency syndrome).

Table 1.1.   Medical history and choice of anaesthesia.

Condition	Clinical problem	Avoiding action
Cardiovascular		
Ischaemic heart disease, angina, myocardial infarction, coronary artery bypass graft	arrhythmias, further ischaemia, GA risk	control pain and anxiety, LA preferred to GA, consider hospital treatment
Congenital heart disease, rheumatic fever, prosthetic heart valve	infective endocarditis	appropriate antibiotic cover
Heart failure	orthopnoea	sit patient up
Thrombo-embolic disease	deep vein thrombosis pulmonary embolus	avoid GA (or give prophylaxis against DVT)
Respiratory		
Asthma	acute asthmatic attack	inhaled bronchodilator pre-op, avoid stress (precipitating factor)
Chronic bronchitis Emphysema	GA risk – obstructed airways –post-op chest infection	use LA
Cystic fibrosis Fibrosing alveolitis	GA risk – restricted lung volume – poor lung function	use LA
Nervous system		
Epilepsy	fits during treatment	maintain anticonvulsive medication
Cerebrovascular accident (CVA) (stroke)	further CVA, potential GA risk	use LA, control anxiety
Multiple sclerosis	exacerbation of MS	avoid GA if possible
Gastro-intestinal		
Peptic ulcer	gastro-intestinal haemorrhage	avoid aspirin and non-steroidal anti-inflammatory drugs
Liver failure	haemorrhage impaired drug metabolism	check prothrombin time adjust drug dosage
Inflammatory bowel disease Malabsorption conditions	steroid therapy (steroid crisis) anaemia (potential GA risk)	give steroid cover LA preferred
Haematological		
Clotting/platelet disorders Anticoagulant therapy	excessive bleeding	liaise with physician correct deficiency/reduce drug
Anaemias, esp. sickle cell	GA risk impaired wound healing	use LA boost haemoglobin level
White cell disorders	infection risk	meticulous sterility, prophylactic antibiotics
Endocrine		
Diabetes mellitus	hyper- or hypoglycaemia nil by mouth for GA	monitor blood glucose level LA preferred
Adrenal/pituitary disease Steroid therapy	steroid (Addisonian) crisis	give steroid cover
Hyperthyroidism	arrythmias thyroid crisis	avoid adrenaline in LA avoid GA/?postpone surgery

Table 1.1. (continued)

Condition	Clinical problem	Avoiding action
Hypothyroidism	slow drug metabolism	LA preferred
	Genito-urinary	
Pregnancy	teratogenicity	avoid surgery in first trimester
	premature labour	avoid third trimester
Renal failure	impaired drug excretion, platelet function reduced, anaemia, cross-infection risk	careful drug/dose selection, liaise with physician, hospital treatment preferred
Renal transplant	immunosuppressive therapy	hospital treatment

LA, local anaesthetic; GA, general anaesthetic.

3. Ischaemic heart disease – recent myocardial infarction (within 3 months), unstable angina.

There is a further group of patients whose treatment is better undertaken in hospital under controlled conditions with full emergency back-up facilities:

1. High risk patients for infective endocarditis such as those with prosthetic heart valves.
2. Patients who have had previous radiotherapy to the jaws and are at risk of osteoradionecrosis (see Chapter 5).

Choice of anaesthesia

Surgical factors

The factors influencing the choice of anaesthetic technique include the aspects of the patient's medical history and their anticipated level of co-operation, as discussed above. Indeed these factors may dictate that a general anaesthetic is required irrespective of the surgical task. However, there are a variety of surgical factors that may indicate the use of local or general anaesthesia.

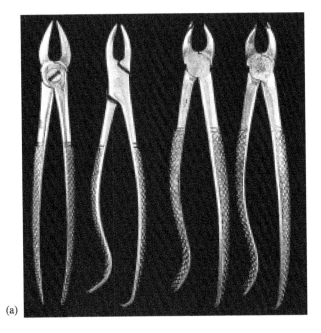

(a)

Figure 1.18. (a) Extraction forceps for upper teeth – from left to right – upper straight forceps, upper premolar forceps (Read pattern), upper right molar forceps and upper left molar forceps.

Local anaesthesia is best for:

- procedures taking less than 30–45 min
- single operative site in the mouth
- readily accessible areas of the mouth.

General anaesthesia is best for:

- complicated procedures of unpredictable duration
- multiple operative sites
- working in areas of the mouth with difficult access (e.g. surgical procedures in the palate).

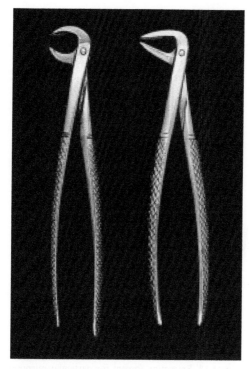

Figure 1.18. (b) Extraction forceps for lower teeth: left – lower molar forceps, right – lower premolar forceps.

INSTRUMENTS

The instrumentation required for simple intra-alveolar extractions can be limited to the basic selection of forceps shown in Figure 1.18a, b. In addition, some forceps for special purposes may be included, but are not essential (Figure 1.19). The detailed description of these forceps and their methods of use are set out in Chapter 2.

For surgical procedures a more extensive array of instruments for raising and replacing soft tissue flaps as well as cutting bone is needed. Conventionally this collection of surgical instruments is laid out as shown in Figure 1.20 on a sterile towel.

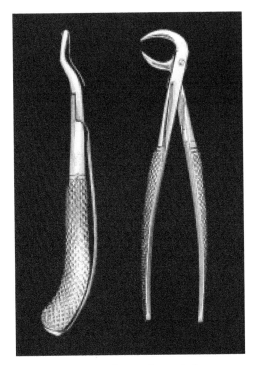

Figure 1.19. Extraction forceps for particular purposes: left – bayonet forceps for upper third molars, right – cowhorn forceps to engage the bifurcation of difficult lower molars.

The set comprises:

1. Scalpel handle, size 3.
2. Number 15 scalpel blade (pre-packed, sterile).
3. Howarth periosteal elevator, with two ends: spatulate (for normal use) and rugine (sharp edge for tough tissue).
4. Ward periosteal elevator (fine spatulate blade for awkward areas).
5. Kilner cheek retractor.
6. Lacks tongue retractor.
7. Bowdler–Henry (rake) flap retractor (also holds back the cheek in the crook of its shank).

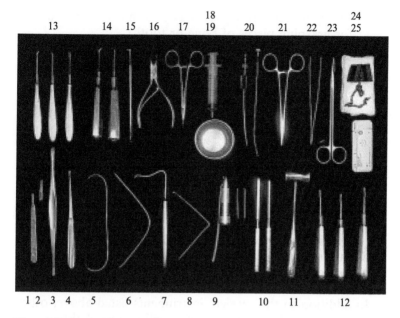

Figure 1.20. Surgical instruments laid out for use – individual instruments identified by number and named in the main text.

8. Austin flap retractor (multipurpose – toothed at one end, plain at the other).
9. Dental handpiece and a selection of sterilized burs, rosehead and fissure.
10. Chisels, width 5 mm and 3 mm (note chisels have a single bevel – like a wood chisel).
11. Surgical mallet (for use only under general anaesthesia).
12. Coupland's elevators, numbers 1, 2 and 3 (for detailed description of elevators and their use see Chapter 3).
13. Warwick–James' elevators, right, left, straight.
14. Cryer's elevators, right, left.
15. Mitchell's osteo-trimmer (sharp spoon at one end, pointed at the other end – hugely useful for retrieval of small fragments of root or bone, and curetting infected soft tissue from sockets).
16. Bone nibblers or rongeurs (sharp edged – for trimming small attached pieces of bone around sockets).

17. Artery forceps (rarely used as a haemostat – but useful for grasping pieces of bone or tooth).
18. Syringe – 10 ml disposable type (for irrigation of the wound with sterile saline).
19. Galley pot.
20. Sucker with fine bore tip and stilette for unclogging the lumen.
21. Needle holder (the jaws are flat for holding needles at varying angles, unlike artery clips which have ridged jaws).
22. Toothed dissecting forceps (for holding the edges of flaps whilst suturing).
23. Scissors (for dissection and cutting sutures).
24. Mouth props (essential for general anaesthesia, sometimes helpful for patients under local anaesthesia).
25. Suture – pre-packed, sterile (braided silk 3/0 gauge on a curved cutting needle is the easiest to use).

In addition to the surgical instruments listed above, other essential items of equipment are a well-focused light source, an adjustable chair and an autoclave; all items present in the dental surgery.

Chapter 2

Intra-alveolar extraction

Dental forceps are used to extract the majority of erupted teeth. These instruments enable the operator to grasp the root of a tooth and exert force directly to the root mass in order to displace it from the surrounding bone. Forceps are designed with relatively short blades (beaks) to engage the tooth root, and relatively longer handles that offer a large mechanical advantage in both gripping and moving the tooth. The potential to apply substantial forces must therefore be appreciated by the operator, as well as the possibility of those forces becoming dangerously excessive.

THE USE OF FORCEPS

Forceps are intended to grasp the roots of teeth, not their crowns. The shape of forceps blades needs therefore to conform to the shape of the root both around its circumference (Figure 2.1) and along its length (Figure 2.2).

Figure 2.1a shows the ideal conformity of blade to root, with contact, and therefore support, over the whole width of the blade. In reality this is unlikely to happen.

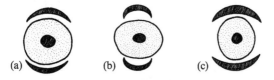

Figure 2.1. (a) Forceps blades with curvature ideal to fit evenly around the circumference of the root. (b) Two point contact of forceps blades on either side of the root. (c) Single point contact on each side of the root.

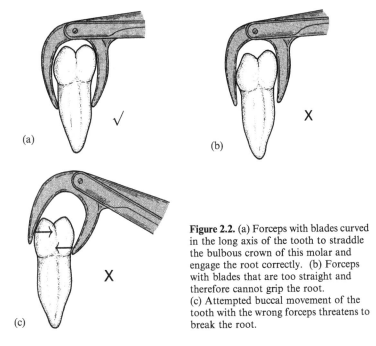

Figure 2.2. (a) Forceps with blades curved in the long axis of the tooth to straddle the bulbous crown of this molar and engage the root correctly. (b) Forceps with blades that are too straight and therefore cannot grip the root.
(c) Attempted buccal movement of the tooth with the wrong forceps threatens to break the root.

Figure 2.1b shows two point contact with a blade more curved and narrower than the root. This arrangement supports the root across the full width of the blade and is the best practical option.

Figure 2.1c demonstrates how blades that are too wide only make a single point contact on each side. Force on the root is concentrated at this point, therefore the risk of root fracture is higher, and a less stable grip results.

Figure 2.2a shows the curvature of the forceps blades in the long axis of the tooth. The blades are seen to straddle the crown and engage the root.

Figure 2.2b demonstrates forceps with insufficient curvature in this plane; the blades are propped apart by the wide crown and unable to engage the relatively narrower root of this molar tooth. As the extraction is attempted, the forceps blades rock to one side as shown in Figure 2.2c and set up a turning moment from the lingual side of the crown to the buccal side of the root. This combination of forces is liable to break the tooth.

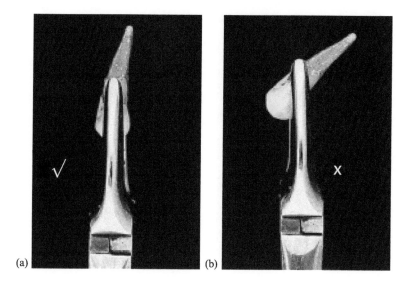

(a)　　　　　　　(b)

Figure 2.3. (a) Correct alignment of forceps blades on the root parallel to its long axis. (b) Poor alignment of forceps blades resulting in inadequate grasp of the root.

Tips of forceps blades should be sharp to facilitate penetration into the periodontal space between the root and surrounding bone. Stainless steel forceps blades can be sharpened on their outer aspect using a sandpaper disc. Blunt, thick blade tips deny the operator any 'feel' whilst the forceps are positioned on the root, and may lead to crushing of surrounding tissues. Entry of the forceps blades into the periodontal space can also be facilitated by first widening the space using a fine elevator.

Application of forceps blades

Forceps blades should be aligned with the long axis of the tooth for extraction to give maximum support and to distribute evenly the forces applied to the root. Malalignment of the forceps may allow the instrument to slip off the root whilst pressure is applied and will concentrate forces at the

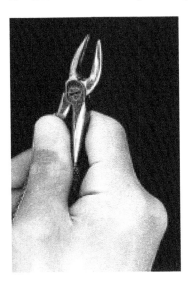

Figure 2.4. Upper straight forceps with fine blades.

points of contact, so increasing likelihood of root fracture. The direction of approach to any given tooth in the mouth with the appropriate forceps is therefore critical (Figure 2.3a, b).

DIFFERENT TYPES OF FORCEPS

Given the basic principles of forceps use above, it can be easily appreciated that a variety of shapes and sizes of forceps is required for different teeth, both because of their varying anatomical form and their position in the mouth. Upper forceps have their handles in line with the blades, whilst the handles of lower forceps are set at right angles to the blades. Blades vary in width, length and curvature to accommodate the different shapes of single-rooted teeth, and those with a single buccal and palatal root such as upper first premolars. Upper molar forceps have blades to fit the two buccal roots and one palatal root of maxillary molar teeth. Mandibular molar teeth have mesial and distal roots and therefore the buccal and lingual blades of lower molar forceps are each shaped to accommodate two roots.

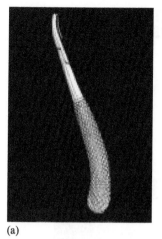

(a)

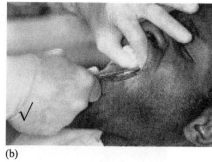

(b)

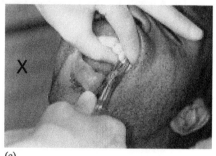

(c)

Figure 2.5. (a) Side view of upper premolar forceps. Note the curvature of the handles in a mesial direction relative to the blades to bring the handles out of the mouth and avoid the lower lip. (b) Upper premolar forceps correctly aligned to engage the first premolar. (c) Inappropriate use of upper straight forceps on a premolar tooth. The handles of the instrument are traumatizing the lower lip

Straight forceps are the simplest design and are suitable for upper incisors and canines. These anterior maxillary teeth are easily accessible using straight-handled forceps, or upper straights, as they are commonly called (Figure 2.4).

Upper premolar forceps have handles that are angled in a mesial direction relative to the blades, thus allowing correct alignment of the blades approaching upper premolar teeth (Figure 2.5a, b), and avoiding the handles fouling the lower teeth or lip, as would happen with straight forceps (Figure 2.5c). *Read* pattern handles have an additional curvature at the ends of the handles to allow this part of the instrument to sit more comfortably in the palm of the hand whilst upward pressure is exerted on the tooth (see Figure 1.18a).

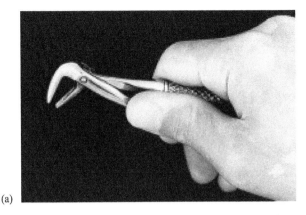

(a)

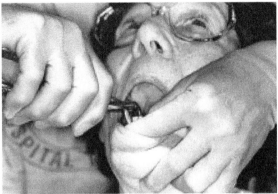

(b)

Figure 2.6. (a) Lower root forceps and the grip for their use. (b) Positioning of lower root forceps on a canine. Note also the stabilization of the jaw with the left hand.

Lower 'root' forceps

As discussed previously, all forceps are designed to engage the roots of teeth to be extracted, but the name 'root forceps' may be given to instruments designed to grasp a single root. All lower forceps are angled with their handles at roughly 90° from their blades, and therefore the handles sit in the axial plane (horizontally if the patient is upright) perpendicular to the dental arch. This allows the optimum position of the operator's hand for both power and control (Figure 2.6a, b).

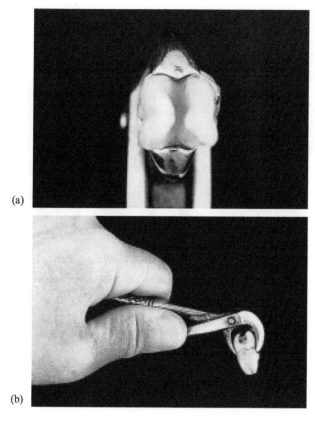

(a)

(b)

Figure 2.7. (a) Twin beaks of lower molar forceps engaging this two-rooted tooth viewed from its apex. (b) Curved blades allow the root to be engaged as the crown is straddled.

Lower molar forceps

Lower first molar teeth normally have two mesial roots, one lingual, one buccal, and a single distal root. In lower second molars, the two mesial roots are often fused, but the distal root remains separate. The root pattern in lower third molars is variable. Most lower molars therefore show two roots when viewed from either the buccal or lingual aspects and so the extraction forceps need a twin beak (blade) on both sides (Figure 2.7a, b). Note that the curvature of the beaks is

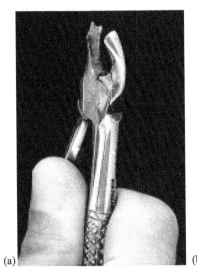

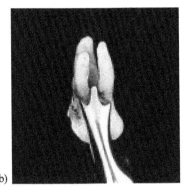

(a)   (b)

Figure 2.8. (a) Upper right molar forceps with a twin beak to engage two buccal roots. (b) The forceps in correct position on an upper right molar tooth.

pronounced to accommodate the bulbous crown and still engage the tooth roots.

All patterns of forceps described so far can be used on either side of the mouth. This bilateral versatility is not true of upper molar forceps.

Upper molar forceps

Maxillary first and second molar teeth generally have two buccal roots and a single palatal root. The forceps are therefore twin beaked on the buccal side and have a single blade palatally. Like upper premolar forceps, the handles are curved in a mesial direction to offer correct alignment of the blades on the tooth with the handle approaching at an angle from the front of the mouth. Because of the offset handles and the asymmetric beaks, the instrument is not reversible and separate forceps are needed for right and left sides. To remember how to identify the right from left forceps, simply think '*beak to cheek*', i.e. twin beak on the buccal side (Figure 2.8a, b).

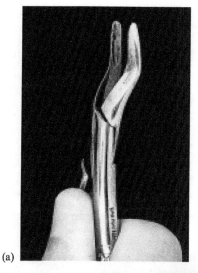

(a)

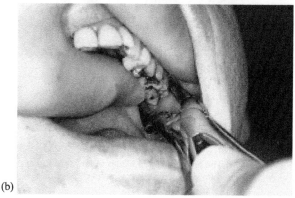

(b)

Figure 2.9. (a) Bayonet forceps with offset blades to reach the posterior maxillary teeth. (b) Bayonet forceps in action on an upper third molar.

Bayonet forceps

Upper third molar teeth may require forceps with additional 'distal reach' for proper alignment of the blades on the root. Bayonet forceps have blades offset substantially in a distal direction for this purpose. The shape resembles a bayonet rifle attachment, hence the name (Figure 2.9a, b).

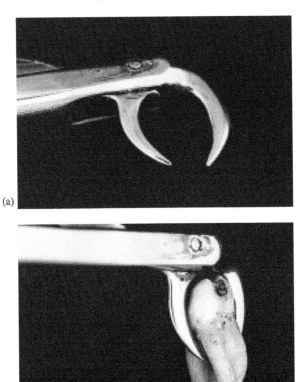

(a)

(b)

Figure 2.10. (a) The pointed curved blades of cowhorn forceps.
(b) A two-rooted lower molar with cowhorns in position.

Other types of forceps

There are many specialized types of forceps designed with
either handles or blades cranked at varying angles and
directions to permit access to teeth in awkward parts of the
mouth. Also there are some with radically modified blades
and one such, 'cowhorn' forceps, can be especially helpful for
difficult lower molars (often the most obstinate teeth to
extract).

Cowhorn forceps (Figure 2.10a, b) have inwardly curved pointed blades designed to engage the furcation of a lower molar tooth when difficulty in gaining a grip on the tooth is found with conventional style forceps. The points of the blades are angled so that as the handles are squeezed together, the blades reach a deeper and more secure hold between the roots.

Forceps for deciduous teeth have narrower, shorter blades designed for the smaller scale of teeth in the primary dentition. Upper 'straights', offset upper 'roots' (like Read forceps), lower 'roots' and lower molar pattern forceps are commonly available.

MECHANICS OF EXTRACTION USING FORCEPS

Positioning the patient is an important but much neglected part of preparation for tooth extraction. By convention, exodontia has been taught with the patient sitting upright in the dental chair. Historically, most dental general anaesthetics were also administered in this position.

In many instances, especially for removal of difficult lower teeth, the upright position is ideal. However, some parts of the mouth are more easily approached by instruments, light and the operator's visual axis with the patient in a supine or semi-recumbent position. This is particularly true of posterior maxillary teeth.

As most operative dentistry is carried out on the supine patient, and all modern equipment is arranged to facilitate this, it seems logical that tooth extraction could also be undertaken in this position. There is undoubtedly some loss of power when the operator is seated as opposed to standing (try throwing a ball from a standing or sitting position and see which goes further). Whilst the importance of controlled power should not be underestimated (see later – moving the tooth), there may be enhanced comfort for both patient and dentist with the supine/seated arrangement. Whichever position is chosen, the patient's head needs to be adequately and comfortably supported by the headrest portion of the chair.

Most dentists prefer to use extraction forceps only in their dominant hand. Further description will therefore apply to holding forceps in the right hand with the assumption that left-handed or ambidextrous operators will make the appropriate changes.

Positioning the operator

Good access to the extraction site is the principal goal in positioning both the patient and the operator. With the patient sitting up, all areas of the mouth are accessible from the right side of the patient. For all upper teeth and those in the lower left quadrant, a stance in front of the patient is best, while for extractions in the lower right quadrant, the operator should stand slightly behind the patient (Figure 2.11a, b).

The height of the patient is important relative to the operator. For lower extractions the target tooth should be at the level of the operator's elbow, and for extraction of upper teeth it is better either to raise the chair to put the tooth nearer shoulder height, or to lean the patient back a little and stand slightly further away (towards the patient's feet). These adjustments maximize both ease of access and mechanical effectiveness. Extracting teeth is a job for the large muscle groups of the legs, trunk and shoulders (for explanation see later – moving the tooth). Standing too close encourages wristy movements which are apt to fracture roots.

With the patient supine, and considering the dental chair as a clock face with the head at 12 o'clock, both upper quadrants are accessible from a seated position to the right of the patient at 7 o'clock. The lower right quadrant is comfortably reached from the operator's chair positioned at 11 o'clock, whilst access to the lower left anterior teeth (incisors and canine) is best from the 10 o'clock position. Approach to the posterior lower teeth on the left requires the operator either to lean across the patient from the right at 7 o'clock or, more logically, to change places with the dental

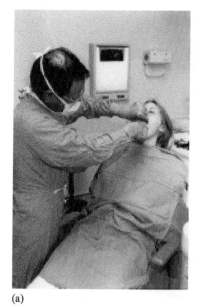
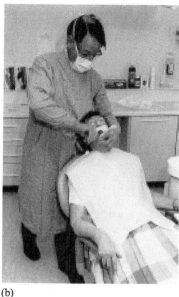

(a)   (b)

Figure 2.11. (a) Access to the upper jaw – approach from the front with the patient's head at the height of the operator's shoulder. (b) Approach to the lower jaw – from behind with the patient's head at the operator's elbow height.

surgery assistant and sit to the left of the patient at 4 o'clock (Figure 2.12a, b).

Gripping the forceps

The importance of gripping the forceps properly cannot be overstated. The ends of the handles should be against the heel of the hand so that pressure along the long axis of the instrument to the tooth is powerful and secure.

The right thumb is placed just below the hinge to help control the width of the blades as the handles are gently squeezed together or moved apart by the fingers. Note the position of the little finger on the inside of the handles in Figure 2.13 as it is used to widen the handles as the forceps are adjusted whilst being placed on the tooth for extraction.

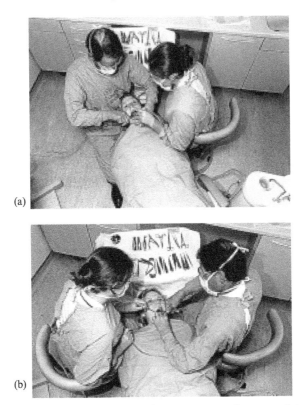

Figure 2.12. (a) Patient supine, operator seated – approach to the lower right quadrant. (b) Access to the lower left quadrant with the patient supine.

The little finger should then be moved to outside the handles as the tooth is gripped ready for displacement. Controlling the distance between the blades of the forceps is difficult for the inexperienced operator, and a helpful exercise to practise is to pick up a pencil from a desk top using lower root forceps, gently holding the pencil without crushing it. Replacing the pencil onto the desk requires delicately releasing the pressure on the handles and then opening the blades with the use of the little finger as described above. The thumb helps to control this fine movement. Repeating the exercise over and over will quickly give the feel of placing the forceps blades into the correct position to grasp the tooth

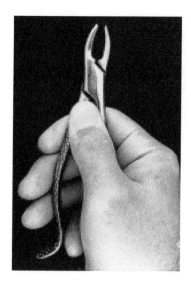

Figure 2.13. The grip for upper forceps.

root without damaging the surrounding tissues.

The left hand also has a vital role to play in supporting the alveolus at the extraction site. In this way the jaw is stabilized so that movements with the forceps do not merely move the whole head or cause displacement or even dislocation of the mandible (see Figure 2.6b). Significant force applied with dental forceps is uncomfortable for the patient unless sufficient support is provided. At the same time the fingers and thumb of the left hand retract the lips, cheeks or tongue to allow free access to the extraction site.

Applying forceps to the tooth

With the left hand retracting the soft tissues out of harm's way, and the forceps gripped correctly in the right hand, the forceps blades are applied carefully to the tooth root. The blades must penetrate into the periodontal space between the root and the alveolar bone (Figure 2.14) and reach as far towards the root apex as possible in order to achieve a stable grip on the root. This positioning of the forceps is crucial to the success of the procedure and warrants care being taken.

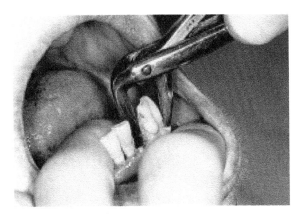

Figure 2.14. Blades of the forceps penetrating the plane between root and alveolar bone.

Time spent at this stage is never wasted. One side of the tooth (usually the lingual or palatal) is often less accessible, and therefore more difficult for forceps placement, and it is prudent to place the more difficult side of the forceps first. A carious cavity or large restoration may similarly complicate forceps extraction.

Once the blades of the forceps are in the correct plane between the root and bone, force is directed parallel to the long axis of the root to drive as far apically as can be reasonably achieved (Figure 2.15a, b). The root is gripped firmly but not crushed, then movements to begin tooth displacement can start. In the case of a multi-rooted molar, the choice of full molar forceps allows the whole root mass to be grasped, provided that the wide blades can penetrate the periodontal space. If good access is not achieved using molar forceps, an alternative strategy is to select finer bladed root forceps that can be worked into better position on the root. The single blade must be applied to one root on each side of the tooth and not pushed into the bifurcation where neither root would be adequately supported (Figure 2.16).

An exception to this general rule is when using cowhorn forceps that are intended to engage the furcation of a difficult lower molar and often split the roots apart, enabling the separate fragments to be elevated more easily.

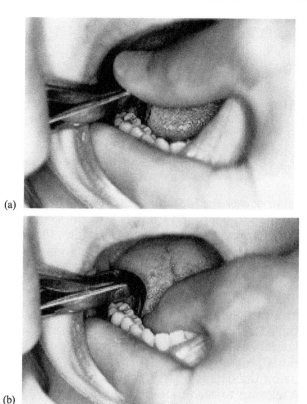

(a)

(b)

Figure 2.15. (a) Thumb of the left hand exerting downward force to drive the forceps apically along the root. (b) With the forceps in position the alveolus is stabilized with the left hand before moving the tooth.

Moving the tooth

Extracting teeth requires the use of controlled force. The tooth is displaced by progressively expanding its bony socket with smooth but positive effort. Rapid, jerky movement is more likely to fracture the tooth than to loosen its root. Such smooth controlled power can only be delivered by the large muscle groups of the shoulders, back and legs. Wristy movements and exclusive use of forearms will quickly tire these smaller muscles whereupon the operator senses failure and resorts to a desperate tugging action that is either

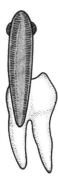

Figure 2.16. Diagram showing the correct placement of fine forceps blades on teeth with more than one root.

ineffectual or causes the tooth to break. Power from the large muscles of the shoulders and trunk is brought to bear on the forceps by fixing the wrist, elbow and shoulder, then moving the whole body from the waist (if sitting) or from the legs (if standing). Considerable control of this applied force can then be exercised by using a small proportion of the potential power of muscles that are also less prone to fatigue.

It must also be appreciated that most teeth in the mouth are not pulled out but pushed out. Apical pressure combined with a lateral (usually predominantly buccal) or rotational movement is generally the best basic strategy, but there are variations on the details of technique according to the local anatomy relevant to each tooth in the jaws.

Direction to move teeth for extraction

Exodontia is an art that must be learned and the operator gaining experience will begin to appreciate the 'feel' of each tooth as it moves and so exploit the line of least resistance. There are, however, some rules for each tooth based on the root form and the local bony anatomy of the alveolus.

Maxillary teeth

Bone in the maxilla has a higher proportion of cancellous to cortical structure than the mandible and as a result is generally less dense than mandibular bone. The alveolar bone

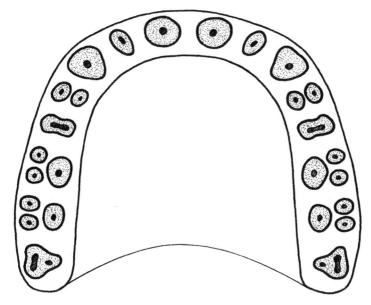

Figure 2.17. Typical root pattern of upper teeth shown in cross-section at mid-root level.

is thinner on its buccal or labial surface by comparison with the thicker palatal side. Therefore the normal direction of tooth displacement is buccally. However, the buccal plate of bone is buttressed in the first molar region by the zygomatic process of the maxilla.

The number and shape of roots materially affect the way in which a tooth is removed. Figure 2.17 shows the typical root pattern of the adult upper dentition seen in axial (horizontal) cross-section.

Table 2.1 gives the root pattern of maxillary teeth related to the direction of displacement using dental forceps.

Technique for individual maxillary teeth

Central incisors normally have a straight conical shaped root with a circular cross-section that yields to primary rotation with upper straight forceps.

Table 2.1. Direction of movement for maxillary teeth.

Tooth in maxilla	Root pattern	Movement
Central incisor	conical – circular cross-section	rotation
Lateral incisor	oval cross-section – flattened mesio-distally	buccal + gentle rotation
Canine	long thick root – triangular cross-section	buccal
First premolar	two thin roots – very fragile – buccal + palatal	wiggle and pull, only tooth in mouth to pull out
Second premolar	one generally strong root	buccal
First molar	two thin buccal roots, one strong palatal root – three roots diverge markedly	buccal – predominantly disto-buccal twist to deliver
Second molar	normally three roots as for first molar	buccal – disto-buccal twist
Third molar	roots very variable	buccal – disto-buccal twist

Lateral incisors   have a straight but slender root that is oval in cross-section, being flattened mesio-distally. Fine-bladed forceps should be used and pushed well up the root to give it support before moving it carefully in a buccal direction.

Canines   have a sturdy root somewhat triangular in cross-section and longer than adjacent teeth. Consequently, removal of the canine may be difficult and not infrequently results in fracture of the labial plate of bone which is then removed with the root. When extracting several adjacent maxillary teeth including the canine, it is advisable to remove the canine before the lateral incisor or the first premolar as the loss of these teeth will weaken further the labial plate of bone. Alternatively, stubborn canines may be safely removed using a surgical (or trans-alveolar) approach.

First premolars   almost universally have two slender roots that are easily fractured. Special care should be taken to position the blades of fine Read forceps high up the roots which must then be dislodged by gently wiggling the tooth in a bucco-palatal direction whilst *pulling*. This is the only tooth in the mouth which is pulled out, not pushed. Moving the roots too far laterally often results in fracture of one (usually the buccal) which then may need to be retrieved by dissection.

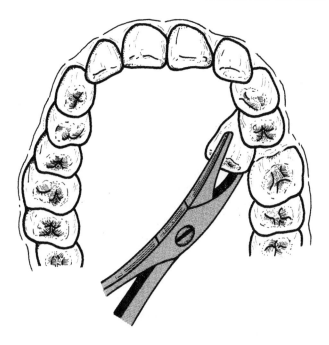

Figure 2.18. Upper premolar forceps placed mesio-distally across an instanding second premolar in the palate.

Second premolars normally have a stout single root, oval in cross-section, that can safely be displaced in a buccal direction. This tooth is, however, often crowded out of the dental arch to an instanding position palatally so that buccal movement is prevented (Figure 2.18). It may still be possible to grip the tooth with fine forceps placed mesio-distally and dislodge it with antero-posterior movement and careful rotation. If this fails then a surgical approach is required, raising a palatal flap to permit the bone obstructing tooth movement to be removed.

First molars usually have one palatal and two buccal roots; all three may diverge widely. Upper molar forceps should be pushed well up onto the root mass before dislodging the tooth with buccal movements whilst maintaining upward pressure. If the tooth is resistant, patience is required to expand the socket gently but positively until further loosening of the tooth is achieved. The delivery is achieved by 'rolling' the tooth out over the buccal plate of bone. For the right maxillary molars the operator should lower his or her right shoulder to effect this rolling movement, and raise the shoulder for upper left molars. In this way a controlled and progressive displacing force is maintained without the wristy snatches that lead to tooth fracture.

Second molars   may have a variable root pattern that is often angled obliquely to the crown and is therefore difficult to grasp effectively with full molar forceps; premolar forceps are preferable in this circumstance, with the blade on the buccal side being engaged on one of the buccal roots but not between them (see Figure 2.16).

Third molars   often have a single conical root but may also have multiple roots, three, four or even five in number. The crown of this last standing maxillary molar is normally inclined slightly disto-angularly so that the crown is placed further distal than the roots, making placement of the forceps awkward. Additional difficulty with access is caused by the presence of the coronoid process of the mandible as the mouth is opened. Try putting the tip of your little finger buccal to your own upper last molar and then open your mouth widely and feel how the coronoid process encroaches to displace the finger. With the mouth halfway open and the chin moved across towards the side of the extraction, there is much more space available.

Proximity of the maxillary antrum

When extracting any maxillary tooth from the first premolar (or even the canine) anteriorly to the last molar posteriorly, the operator needs to be aware of the close anatomical relationship of the maxillary antrum just above the apices of these teeth. This is particularly relevant with difficult molar teeth, especially the wisdom tooth which often fails to erupt fully. Occasionally the bone separating the tooth roots from

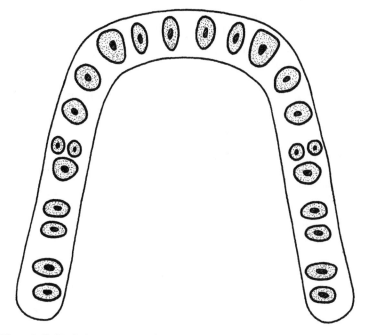

Figure 2.19. Typical root pattern of lower teeth shown in cross-section at mid-root level.

the nasal sinus is very thin and may be fractured, leaving a communication that may become an established fistula between the tooth socket and the sinus (see section on oro – antral fistula in Chapter 5). When the possibility of antral involvement is suspected, it is often safer to remove the tooth using a surgical approach.

Mandibular teeth

The mandible has a higher ratio of cortical to cancellous bone than the maxilla. Consequently the alveolar bone supporting lower teeth is more dense and less readily deformed, making the displacement of mandibular teeth more difficult, particularly the molars. Buccal and lingual cortices tend to be of similar thickness in the anterior mandible. Further distally, in the second and third molar regions, the buccal plate of bone is thickened by the external oblique ridge. Figure 2.19 shows the root pattern of the lower teeth seen in cross-section in the axial (horizontal) plane.

Table 2.2 describes the typical root form of mandibular teeth related to the direction of displacement with dental forceps.

Table 2.2. Directions of movement for mandibular teeth.

Tooth in mandible	Root pattern	Movement
Central + lateral incisors	thin oval cross-section – flattened mesio-distally	bucco-lingual
Canine	long thick root – triangular cross-section	bucco-lingual
First and second premolars	round cross-section	rotation
First molar	two mesial roots, one distal	bucco-lingual – figure of 8
Second molar	normally as for first molar	lingual–buccal – figure of 8
Third molar	root pattern very variable	lingual – figure of 8

Technique for individual mandibular teeth

Lower incisors have fine roots that are flattened mesio-distally, making their bucco-lingual profile very narrow and necessitating the use of fine-bladed lower root forceps. These teeth normally yield to gentle bucco-lingual movement, but their roots may be fragile and do break easily. When removing several adjacent teeth, a useful technique is first to loosen them with a narrow straight elevator such as a Coupland's number 1 or a straight Warwick–James. Figure 2.20a, b demonstrates the technique of loosening two adjacent teeth prior to forceps extraction. N.B. this technique is only appropriate when both teeth are to be removed (see also section on use of elevators later in this chapter).

Canines have a longer, thicker root than lower incisors or premolars and require heavier bladed forceps. If the root is

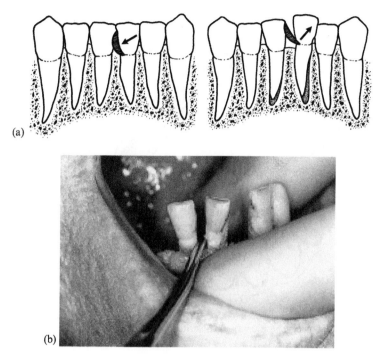

Figure 2.20. Diagram (a) and photograph (b) of an elevator tip loosening a tooth using the adjacent tooth (also for extraction at the same visit) as a fulcrum.

resistant to buccal movement combined with a little judicious secondary rotation, then a surgical approach is indicated and is preferable to the retrieval of a fractured root.

First and second premolars usually have a straight single root that is round in cross-section and therefore amenable to displacement by primary rotation. The operator must appreciate however that lower forceps (which have handles at right angles to the blades) offer a huge mechanical advantage in a rotational movement, rather like a screwdriver with a T-piece handle. Therefore care must be taken not to force the movement or a spiral fracture of the root will result. Lower second premolars are not uncommonly crowded out of the arch lingually, or may be impacted in the alveolus between the first premolar and molar. The lingually placed

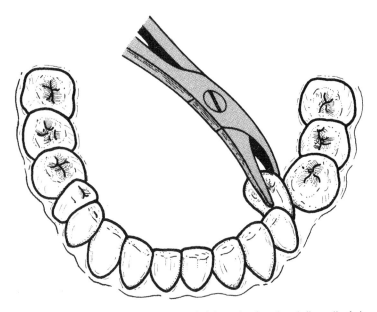

Figure 2.21. Lower second premolar excluded from the dental arch lingually, being grasped mesio-distally with upper premolar forceps.

tooth may be grasped using upper premolar forceps applied mesio-distally from across the arch (Figure 2.21). Impacted lower second premolars can be among the most difficult and demanding teeth to remove and normally require a surgical procedure (see Chapter 3).

Lower first molars classically have two mesial roots, one buccal, one lingual, and a single distal root. Lower molar forceps with their broad twin beaks both lingually and buccally grasp the whole of this root mass. Sometimes these forceps are difficult to apply satisfactorily when the alveolar bone is very dense, or if the tooth has a carious cavity or large restoration at the cervical margin. A different strategy is to use lower root forceps, aiming to place the blades low down on either the mesial roots or the distal root (see Figure 2.16). Alternatively, cowhorn forceps, with their pointed blades, can be worked into the bifurcation from both buccal and lingual aspects.

Movement of the lower first molar should be principally towards the buccal side with bucco-lingual oscillation and 'figure of 8' movements to expand the socket (Figure 2.22).

The root may then be 'rolled' out over the buccal plate of bone. If the lingual wall of the tooth is deficient or weakened by caries, primary movement should be towards the lingual side as forceful buccal displacement is likely either to fracture the tooth, or the forceps blades will merely slip out of position.

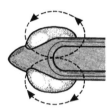

Figure 2.22. Diagram to show 'figure of 8' movements to displace a lower molar.

Lower second molars have a root pattern similar to the lower first molar except that the two mesial roots are often fused. The buccal plate of alveolar bone becomes thicker distally in the second, and especially the third molar region, and forms the oblique ridge of the mandible. Buccal displacement of second molars may therefore be difficult, and primary movement in a lingual direction is often more fruitful.

Lower third molars (*wisdom teeth*)   show extreme variation in shape and size. As the last tooth to erupt in the lower dentition, they often become impacted due to inadequate space in the dental arch. Even fully erupted third molars can be very difficult to extract as they tend to be encased in dense bone at the base of a concavity (compare with the upper third molar that is normally much easier to dislodge, being at the apex of a convex tuberosity in less dense maxillary bone). The close proximity of the inferior alveolar nerve to the apices of lower wisdom teeth, and the lingual nerve which is immediately adjacent to the mandible in the third molar region, add to the hazards of removing these teeth. A pre-operative radiographic view of the whole tooth with its surrounding structures (inferior dental canal, adjacent tooth, anterior aspect of the mandibular ramus) is mandatory. If forceps extraction is attempted, the primary movement should be towards the lingual side with bucco-lingual rocking and 'figure of 8' rotations to expand the socket. Bone removal is often required, and such a 'surgical' approach should be planned carefully, with appropriate pre-operative information and warnings about potential complications given to the patient. Unanticipated problems, including damage to the lingual or inferior dental nerve, are all too commonly the subjects of litigation.

Deciduous teeth

In general, teeth in the primary dentition are easier to remove than their permanent successors. Deciduous teeth have less substantial roots that are often significantly resorbed. However there are several factors which may detract from this generalization.

The underlying developing permanent tooth   is closely related to the roots of the deciduous tooth and could be damaged by the placement of extraction forceps. This is particularly true in the case of deciduous molars (Figure 2.23). The use of root forceps can simplify gaining a satisfactory grip on fine deciduous roots, but note that the blades must be placed on either the mesial or the distal root and not between them where the permanent tooth may be disturbed.

Fragility of deciduous roots.   Resorption of deciduous roots is not a uniform process from apex to crown. Thin and fragile remnants of roots often result from asymmetric resorption if the permanent tooth erupts slightly to one side of its deciduous counterpart. The fracture of such roots during their extraction may be inevitable. Furthermore, it may be advisable to leave these root fragments to be shed or resorb naturally rather than to risk damage to the permanent tooth by invasive instrumentation. If removal of a retained root

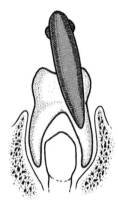

Figure 2.23. Correct placement of forceps on a deciduous molar showing the close proximity of the crown of the underlying permanent tooth.

fragment is considered necessary then a mucoperiosteal flap should be raised, to enable the operator to see the relationship of the root to the permanent tooth, and the procedure conducted under direct vision. Uneven resorption of upper deciduous molar roots often leaves the buccal roots longer than the palatal root and particularly susceptible to fracture if the tooth is moved solely towards the buccal side. In this case the initial displacement should be in a palatal direction in order to loosen the slim buccal roots before delivering the tooth buccally.

Carious crown. Those deciduous teeth needing extraction, particularly molars, often have their crowns broken down with caries. There may be little solid tooth structure above the gingivae which may grow over the remaining root, making accurate placement of the forceps blades between the root and the alveolar bone very difficult. Retraction of the excess gingival tissue with the blades as the forceps are applied will help in visualizing the correct plane, but the careful use of an elevator may be preferable in this circumstance (Figure 2.24).

Restricted access. A child's mouth offers limited surgical access simply because it is small. Placing a mouth prop can help to maximize the available space and may be used whether the patient has general or local anaesthesia. A prop is normally tolerated very well by the conscious patient as it

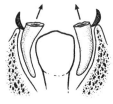

Figure 2.24. Use of Warwick–James' elevator to remove deciduous roots straddling the crown of a lower premolar.

obviates the need for sustained effort, by both patient and operator, to keep the mouth open.

Once the factors listed above have been recognized, the basic technique of extracting deciduous teeth does not differ markedly from that used for permanent teeth and the forceps designed for deciduous teeth are suitably scaled down in size. Displacement of these teeth is normally simply achieved but some molars with unresorbed roots may present a slightly greater challenge. Occasionally such a tooth is surprisingly resistant. This may be due to the tooth becoming ankylosed to the alveolar bone, whereupon the tooth appears to submerge slowly as further appositional growth of the mandible in adjacent areas increases the height of the alveolus. The ankylosed tooth does not move upwards with the rest of the dentition and is thus left in infra-occlusion. Beware such teeth as they will be difficult or impossible to extract without sufficient bone removal following the raising of a mucoperiosteal flap (Figure 2.25).

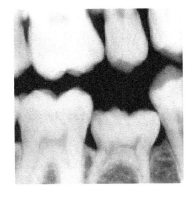

Figure 2.25. Lower deciduous molar sub-merging due to ankylosis of its roots.

Extracting teeth from a crowded arch

When the teeth are irregularly positioned due to crowding, gaining access with extraction forceps is made more difficult and the risk of damaging adjacent teeth is increased. The upper canines and the upper and lower second premolars are commonly excluded from the dental arch as they are the last teeth to erupt in those areas of the jaws. Applying forceps to such a tooth may require the blades to be positioned mesio-distally as shown in Figure 2.18. Fine Read forceps are best, irrespective of which jaw is being approached. The possible direction of displacement may also be severely limited, with small movements and great patience being required. Often these teeth demand a surgical, trans-alveolar approach.

ELEVATORS – THE PRINCIPLES OF USE

Elevators differ fundamentally from forceps in the manner they enable force to be applied to a tooth. Forceps allow the operator to grasp the tooth and apply a force directly to that tooth in the jaw. The same force is thereby also transmitted to the jaw, and the operator's left hand must stabilize the jaw by resisting the displacing movement. An elevator applies force *between* the tooth and the surrounding bone of the jaw. There is therefore no resultant force tending to move the jaw.

Elevators exert less directional control on the tooth than forceps. In this way a root being elevated tends to move along its own path of withdrawal, and may therefore be less likely to fracture, whereas forceps dictate the direction of movement.

Elevators can be thought of as acting like wedges with one side of the wedge applying the force to the tooth at the *point of application* whilst the other side of the wedge applies an equal and opposite force to the adjacent bone – *the fulcrum*. Without either an effective point of application or fulcrum, there is no effective elevation. Also, to be efficient, the elevator tip needs to be of suitable size. A thick wedge will not gain access to a thin space, and if too wide, the tip will merely jam at the first rotatory movement (Figure 2.26a). A tip that is too narrow will rotate round and round in a large space without engaging root or bone and thus achieves nothing (Figure 2.26b). Choice of the correct sized elevator will enable the displacement of a root without excessive lateral force (Figure 2.26c).

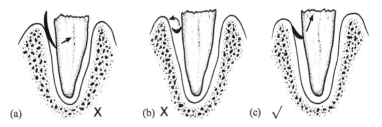

(a)   (b)   (c)

Figure 2.26. (a) Wide elevator in a small space – the direction of displacement is too horizontal and the root is jammed against the bone. (b) Narrow elevator in a large space – nothing is achieved. (c) Correct sized elevator exerting coronal displacing force.

Elevators can also be used to facilitate extraction with forceps by:

- breaking down the periodontal attachment
- allowing access to the forceps at a more apical level
- expanding the bony socket.

When used in this way, there is no attempt to provide any displacing force on the tooth with the elevators, but solely to enable more effective application of the forceps.

Safe use of elevators

The fulcrum for elevation should always be on bone. It is permissible for an adjacent tooth to be used as a fulcrum only if that tooth is also to be extracted at the same session. This technique can be usefully exploited during a dental clearance. Failure to observe this rule may result in damage to, or even inadvertent extraction of, an adjacent tooth. This is

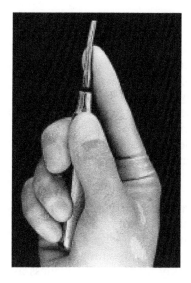

Figure 2.27. Coupland's 'elevator' – how to hold it safely and effectively.

particularly likely if an elevator is engaged interproximally between a large rooted tooth such as a first molar and a smaller rooted second premolar with the aim of dislodging the molar. The equal and opposite reaction on the smaller rooted premolar may be enough to cause its displacement or fracture.

Elevators, like forceps blades, need to be guided carefully but positively into the periodontal space around the root. Unlike forceps, the tip of an elevator can gain access to almost any point around the circumference of the root. Holding the instrument correctly is of paramount importance if the effort of positioning the elevator tip in this way is to be controlled safely (Figure 2.27). The butt of the handle should be in the heel of the hand to provide force parallel to the long axis of the instrument. The index finger is extended down the shaft towards the tip to control the direction of placement and to act as a safety stop should the elevator slip. The thumb and remaining fingers grasp the handle and provide the rotational component of force. It is the rotation movement that allows controlled force to be applied to the tooth root; elevators should never be used as class 1 levers.

Patterns of elevators

Coupland's 'elevators' (see Figure 2.27) were originally designed as chisels, or more accurately, gouges (which are curved at the cutting end). However they make excellent elevators especially when the edges of the tips are sharp and grip well on the root surface. There are three standard widths of tip denoted 1, 2 and 3, with 1 being the narrowest. Generally it is advisable to select the smallest size that is effective, and progress to wider ones as the root becomes loosened.

Warwick–James' elevators have either a straight pattern or a curved tip. The straight Warwick–James' is like a fine Coupland's but without the sharp edges to the tip. It has a narrow, pointed end which is very good at gaining access into tight application points, but quickly loses its effectiveness as the tooth starts to move and the working space between root and bone opens up. When this happens it is tempting to use the elevator as a class 1 lever (like a tyre lever), but this is not advisable as it would result in huge forces being applied due to the mechanical advantage achieved.

Curved Warwick–James' enable the application of a force in a direction almost at right angles to the handle, and like the straight pattern, the tip is fine enough to burrow into small spaces. The tip is angled to the right or left side (Figure 2.28a) and the two are not interchangeable by simply reversing the instrument as the angled tips are themselves curved to give a convex, blunt side and a concave, sharp side. Left can be distinguished from right by holding the instrument with the convex curve of the tip facing the operator. In this position the left Warwick–James' has its angled tip pointing to the left.

Cryer's elevators are a similar shape to curved Warwick–James' but are larger and with a sharp pointed tip (Figure 2.28b). This allows the tip to be advanced through thin alveolar bone with modest hand pressure. Like Warwick–James' elevators, Cryer's have the angled point at slightly less than right angles to the shaft (see Figure 2.28b). Note that these instruments have maximum effect when the angled tip is

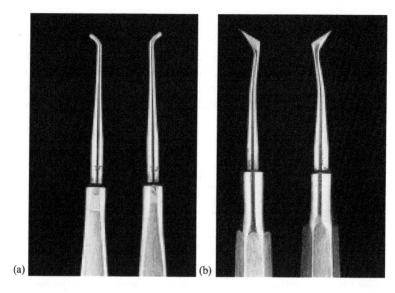

(a)   (b)

Figure 2.28. (a) Warwick–James' elevators, left and right. (b) Cryer's elevators, left and right.

at 90° to the long axis of the tooth rather than when the shaft is parallel to it.

The reader will have appreciated that there is a choice of different elevators for different tasks according to:

- the amount of space available
- the position and availability of a solid fulcrum on *bone*
- the position of a strong application point on the root
- the direction of movement required.

The direction of movement most likely to be effective depends largely on the shape of the root to be elevated. A root with a curvature distally (Figure 2.29a) requires an application point mesially to roll it distally along the path of withdrawal of the root. The exact opposite will pertain for a mesially curved root (Figure 2.29b), whilst a straight, conical root may respond to an application point anywhere on its circumference, the buccal aspect normally being the most easily accessible (Figure 2.29c).

In multi-rooted teeth, the individual roots may point in different directions and thus be resistant to movement along a mean path of withdrawal. If such a tooth cannot be dislodged using extraction forceps, simple elevation is unlikely to succeed and a surgical approach is indicated as either bone removal, division of the tooth, or both of these may be required.

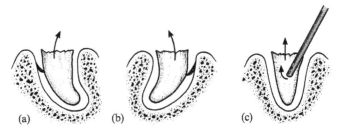

Figure 2.29. Three roots with varying directions of curvature showing the position of effective application points.

POST-EXTRACTION CARE

Checking the socket   following delivery of the tooth ensures that no debris such as pieces of bone, fragments of broken filling material or fractured roots have been inadvertently left in the socket. Careful inspection in good light, preferably with suction available, is recommended. Over-enthusiastic prodding in the depth of the socket with a sucker or other instrument should be avoided, as damage to the inferior dental nerve in the mandible or creating an oro–antral communication in the maxilla could result (see Chapter 5 on complications). The walls of the socket should then be squeezed between finger and thumb to reduce any distortion of the alveolus and overlying mucosa.

Establishing haemostasis   is a top priority before the patient can be discharged.
    The first stage of wound healing is the cessation of bleeding and the establishment of a stable blood clot. To assist haemostasis a gauze pack is placed over the socket, and the

patient instructed to apply gentle but continuous pressure on it by biting. The pack needs to sit closely over the open socket to be effective and should therefore be placed exactly over the extraction site and not over the adjacent teeth. A bulky pack onto which the patient bites will be trapped at the occlusal level of the teeth and will not therefore occlude the socket as intended. The pack should be left undisturbed in the patient's mouth for at least 10 minutes and the patient encouraged not to talk or open the mouth during this time.

Rest in the immediate post-operative phase means sitting quietly until haemostasis is achieved. After that, avoidance of demanding physical work or exercise is recommended for the remainder of the day, as such activities may restart the bleeding.

Food and drink should ideally be avoided whilst the numbness from the local anaesthetic persists otherwise the socket may be disturbed or filled with debris. After a few hours the patient may eat and drink, but nothing too hot which could provoke further bleeding, or too tough to chew which could traumatize the socket.

Analgesia is the responsibility of the dental surgeon who should advise or prescribe appropriate post-operative pain relief. Following uncomplicated tooth extraction, an analgesic such as *paracetamol* is normally adequate and is safer than aspirin for routine use. Aspirin offers effective pain relief but has a number of drawbacks for the post-surgical patient including an increase in bleeding time due to decreased platelet aggregation, gastric irritation with an increased likelihood of intestinal haemorrhage in susceptible patients, and a variety of unwanted interactions with other drugs, notably warfarin.

Non-steroidal anti-inflammatory drugs (NSAIDs) like *ibuprofen* have (as their name suggests) anti-inflammatory as well as analgesic properties that are highly desirable in the post-operative setting. Analgesics may also be given pre-operatively so that an effective dose has been absorbed before the local anaesthetic wears off. Despite the fact that these drugs share many of the unwanted side effects of aspirin, including gastric irritation, potentiation of warfarin and possible exacerbation of bronchospasm in asthmatics, ibuprofen is widely used as a first-line analgesic and is available as an 'over the counter' drug.

Opiate derivatives such as codeine and dihydrocodeine are not routinely indicated for post-operative pain. However they have a place in the management of severe or protracted pain in combination with paracetamol (co-codamol or co-dydramol tablets), and these provide a useful alternative painkilling strategy for those patients for whom the NSAIDs are contraindicated, if paracetamol alone is not sufficient. Codeine and dihydrocodeine require a prescription from the dental surgeon.

Some useful analgesic regimens are as follows:

- Paracetamol, 1 g (one tablet = 500 mg), 4 hourly.
- Ibuprofen, 400 mg (tablets vary in strength), 8 hourly.
- Ibuprofen, 400 mg, 8 hourly + paracetamol, 1 g, 4 hourly as required (this combination of drugs is very effective for moderate to severe dental pain).
- Co-codamol (codeine 30 mg + paracetamol 500 mg), one to two tablets, 6 hourly (maximum six tablets in 24 hours).

For *children*, paracetamol is preferred and the dose is appropriately reduced: 50% of adult dose at age 7, 75% of adult dose at age 12. Aspirin is contraindicated for those under 12 years of age because of the risk of Reye's syndrome.

In *pregnancy*, elective procedures are to be avoided when possible. If tooth extraction becomes necessary, paracetamol is usually the analgesic of choice.

Further prescribing information, including contraindications and side effects of the analgesics suitable for dental use, is given in the Dental Practitioner's Formulary (DPF) section at the front of the British National Formulary (BNF). The reader is strongly recommended to refer to this source of information which is relevant, clear, concise and is constantly updated.

Mouth bathing and tooth brushing

The use of warm salt water mouth baths helps to clean and soothe the mouth after surgery. It is also said that the salt water reduces swelling and may help to prevent infection. A teaspoonful of salt is dissolved in a beaker of warm, but not hot, water and used for gentle bathing of the mouth four times a day, starting the day after surgery, and continuing until the discomfort has resolved. Over-enthusiastic swishing of liquids around the mouth is not a good idea and may dislodge the blood clot and predispose to a dry socket (see Chapter 5). Normal tooth brushing should be resumed as soon as comfort permits. Before that time, a balance needs to be struck between allowing the accumulation of debris around the socket and the risk of traumatizing the wound.

Chapter 3

Trans-alveolar extraction

Some teeth are unsuitable for removal using forceps and the technique of intra-alveolar extraction described in Chapter 2. This may be evident on assessment of the tooth pre-operatively, or may become so during the course of attempted extraction. By adopting the trans-alveolar or 'surgical' approach, the operator gains direct access to the alveolar bone and tooth roots after raising the overlying soft tissues as a mucoperiosteal flap. Bone removal and sectioning of the tooth or its roots under direct vision are then possible in order to expedite the extraction.

INDICATIONS FOR TRANS-ALVEOLAR EXTRACTION

- Any tooth that is resistant to attempts at intra-alveolar extraction when moderate force is applied.
- Retained roots that cannot either be grasped with forceps or delivered using an elevator.
- Buried or impacted teeth.
- When the bone is dense and unyielding. There is often a history of difficult extractions in such patients.
- Hypercementosed or ankylosed teeth.
- Teeth with abnormalities of shape or size, e.g. gemination or dilaceration of the root.
- Teeth having multiple or unfavourable roots with conflicting paths of withdrawal.
- Any tooth or root close to the maxillary antrum that cannot readily be extracted with forceps or elevated.
- For pre-prosthetic adjustment of bone contour in preparation for dentures, bridges or dental implants.

Careful pre-operative assessment of teeth for extraction, as well as the patients to whom they belong, is the key to embarking on a successful surgical procedure. The reader is reminded to read the sections on assessment, both of teeth and patients, in Chapter 1.

Mucoperiosteal flaps

The main aim of raising a soft tissue flap is to establish adequate surgical access to the alveolar bone and tooth roots beneath. Following bone removal and root elevation, the mucoperiosteal flap must be replaced accurately in order to expedite healing of the wound. These surgical manipulations need to be carried out with the minimum of disruption and risk of damage to surrounding structures. The following basic principles of flap design are therefore universally applicable.

Principles of flap design

Shape of flaps. Flaps can be raised that have two or three sides (Figure 3.1a, b, c), and in some circumstances, a 'flap' with only one side along the gingival margin can offer restricted access to the hard tissues at the crest of the alveolus but this is achieved at the risk of stretching and tearing the soft tissues as they are undermined using a periosteal elevator. Sometimes this allows sufficient access to reach a point of application if no bone removal is required.

Two-sided flaps are made with one incision along the gingival margin and another, called the relieving incision, angled obliquely across the attached buccal gingiva into the lax vestibular mucosa. This design of flap gives adequate access for most trans-alveolar extractions.

Three-sided flaps have a second relieving incision at the distal end of the flap. This pattern allows extra mobilization of the soft tissues and hence greater exposure of the underlying bone and roots of teeth, particularly in an apical

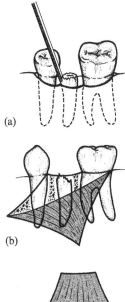

(a)

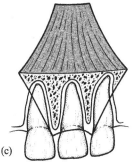

(b)

(c)

Figure 3.1. (a) An incision only along the gingival margin allows very limited access to the superficial part of a root fractured at crestal bone level. (b) Two-sided flap with a mesial relieving incision – this design of flap provides adequate access for most trans-alveolar extractions. (c) Three-sided flap with mesial and distal relieving incisions – this flap improves the access to the apices of teeth.

direction. This type of flap is used to gain access to periapical lesions during apicectomy, and for closure of oro–antral communications by advancement of the flap across the tooth socket (see Chapter 5).

Access is the key to making surgery easy. If you cannot see or reach the target, then any procedure becomes awkward and thus potentially hazardous. Flaps should be large enough to permit clear access to the operation site without the need to stretch, and risk tearing, the soft tissues. An incision 3 cm long heals just as fast as one measuring 1.5 cm!

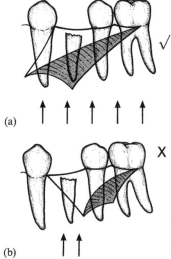

(a)

(b)

Figure 3.2. (a) Correct design of flap with a broad base. (b) Poor flap with narrow base, so restricting blood supply to the flap and limiting access to the buried root.

Blood supply. The base of all flaps should be wider than the free margin to maintain unimpeded blood supply to the tissues of the flap. Figure 3.2a, b shows examples of a well designed flap with a broad base, and a poorly planned flap with an unacceptably narrow base.

Avoiding vital structures. The positioning of relieving incisions must take into account the proximity of important structures, notably the mental nerve which is vulnerable to damage at the mental foramen (Figure 3.3a, b).

Extending flaps. When planning the surgical removal of more than one tooth in the same part of the mouth, a two-sided flap with its relieving incision mesial to the most anterior tooth allows extension in a distal direction as required. Poorly planned and hastily cut flaps may preclude the completion of multiple extractions if more than one requires a surgical approach (Figure 3.4a, b, c). It is also worth remembering that a 'simple' forceps extraction may turn into a surgical procedure requiring a flap to be raised. Therefore when more than one tooth is to be removed, any

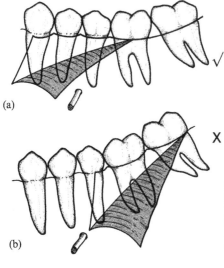

(a)

(b)

Figure 3.3. (a) Correct positioning of relieving incision in the lower premolar region, near the mental foramen. (b) Incorrect site of relieving incision that may damage the mental nerve.

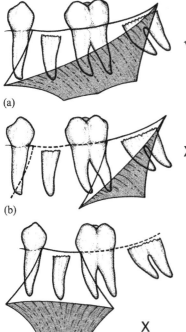

(a)

(b)

(c)

Figure 3.4. (a) Correctly sited flap for removal of roots at lower premolar and molar regions. (b) Incorrect position of relieving incision between the molars preventing extension mesially. (c) Inappropriate use of three-sided flap in the premolar area with the distal relieving incision preventing further distal extension.

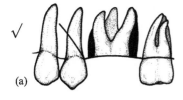

(a)

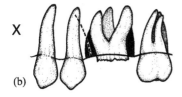

(b)

Figure 3.5. (a) Correct position of incision (and thus the suture line) over intact bone. (b) Incorrect placement of the relieving incision over an area of planned bone removal. This obstructs bone removal and the resulting suture line will be unsupported and lie over a bony cavity.

potentially difficult forceps extractions should be tackled before a decision about flap position is taken.

Suture over bone. The margins of flaps should be placed far enough away from the site of intended bone removal so that the incision lines will be supported by lying over intact bone at the end of the procedure (Figure 3.5a, b).

Ease of closure. Edges of flaps should be positioned to make their accurate replacement simple. Flap margins around teeth should include a whole inter-dental papilla which is then available to be sutured across to the lingual tissues either through the embrasure or at one side of the newly created socket. Starting a relieving incision half way along the crown of a standing tooth prevents such neat closure (see section on suturing later in this chapter).

Closure of an oro–antral communication. Whenever a flap is planned for the removal of a tooth or root in the posterior maxilla, a thought should be given to the possibility of inadvertently creating a communication between the socket and the maxillary sinus. Thus the flap needs to be suitable for closing such a defect, or be capable of modification for this purpose (see Chapter 5).

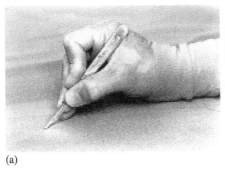

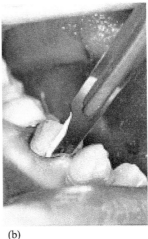

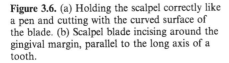

Figure 3.6. (a) Holding the scalpel correctly like a pen and cutting with the curved surface of the blade. (b) Scalpel blade incising around the gingival margin, parallel to the long axis of a tooth.

(a)

(b)

Making the incisions

Incisions are made using a scalpel with a number 15 blade using firm, positive pressure so that all layers of soft tissue from mucosa to periosteum are divided at a single clean, careful stroke. Secondary cuts necessitated by inadequate length or depth of the incision may leave uneven ragged margins to the flap which are difficult to suture and may delay healing. Relieving incisions should always cross the muco–gingival junction to reach the lax tissues of the vestibular mucosa, and so allow the flap to be mobilized easily. However, over-extension of the incision deep into the sulcus may cause excessive haemorrhage from blood vessels within the buccinator muscle, damage to adjacent structures such as the mental nerve, or result in loss of sulcus depth due to scarring.

The scalpel handle is held like a pen, not a plough (Figure 3.6a) and the blade is directed at right angles to the surface of the mucosa so as to produce a neat edge that is not chamfered or undercut. Vertical incisions along the gingival margins of standing teeth require the scalpel to be held parallel to the long axis of the tooth so that the blade sits neatly in the gingival crevice (Figure 3.6b). When such a cleanly cut flap edge is replaced there should be no resulting apical migration of the gingival margin.

Raising the flap

In flaps with two or three sides, the full thickness of the mucoperiosteum is elevated from the underlying bone by introducing the sharp, flat end of a periosteal elevator under the anterior edge of the flap where the relieving incision is through the vestibular mucosa, not the attached gingiva (Figure 3.7). Starting to raise the flap in the tightly bound down gingival tissue is unnecessarily difficult. The periosteum is also tightly adherent to bone over the crest of the alveolar ridge in edentulous spaces, and along the muco–gingival junction where the flap is also most vulnerable to tearing.

Having identified the correct plane of separation at the subperiosteal level, the bone surface is uncovered by advancing the elevation of the flap on a broad front, and not by tunnelling under tissues which may subsequently become stretched or torn. If the flap resists elevation, it is probable that the incision has not divided the periosteum, and this should be rectified before repeated unsuccessful attempts to lift the flap result in damage to its margins. Care needs to be taken to avoid perforating the flap with the relatively sharp end of the periosteal elevator which should be held in contact with the bone surface at all times. The presence of a sinus in the buccal sulcus, when the tooth or root to be removed has a chronic periapical infection, may complicate flap design and elevation, making the flap liable to be 'button holed' (perforated) at this site. By carefully elevating the flap around the sinus opening, the sinus track as it emerges from the bone can be identified and divided with scissors to release the tethered flap without risk of tearing a large hole. Once the source of the infection is removed, the sinus will heal spontaneously. When the flap is raised, it is held well out of the operative field with a suitable retractor, such as the Bowdler–Henry (rake pattern), or the Austin retractor. These instruments serve also to retract the lip or cheek at the same time.

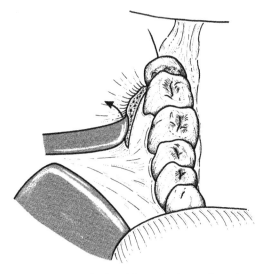

Figure 3.7. The easiest place to begin raising a flap is usually at the margin in loose vestibular mucosa, apical to the muco–gingival junction.

BONE REMOVAL

Bone is a precious commodity in the prosthetic rehabilitation of the jaws even after the teeth it supported have been removed. Bone removal should achieve specific objectives, and not be mindlessly excessive. Before delivery of the tooth or root, bone is removed either:

- to expose the tooth and clear its path of exit
- to provide suitable points of application (see section on use of elevators in Chapter 2).

After the extraction, the dental surgeon may need to trim the walls of the socket:

- to remove any sharp edges
- to smooth the ridge contour to assist the prosthetist.

Instruments for bone removal

Bone can be removed with a dental bur, normally in a straight handpiece, or using chisels or gouges (chisels with curved

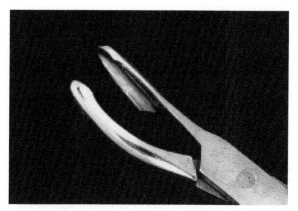

Figure 3.8. Bone nibblers or 'rongeurs' have sharp blades for cutting and trimming bone margins.

cutting ends). Burs are preferred by most dentists because they cut bone predictably and efficiently, provided the bur is sharp. Chisels can peel away soft bone of the maxilla with just hand pressure, but the dense cortical bone in the mandible requires carefully weighted blows with a surgical mallet for the bone surface to be penetrated. This technique is best suited to the experienced operator with the patient under general anaesthesia. Rongeurs, or bone nibblers (Figure 3.8), are useful for trimming prominent or sharp pieces of bone from the margins of the socket once the tooth is out.

Rotary cutting instruments – dental drills and burs

Specialized surgical drills are available on the market with features for optimal bone cutting: high torque at bur speeds of 1000–30 000 revolutions per minute (rpm), and a straight handpiece for maximum control of cutting direction. It is awkward trying to cut bone using a contra-angle handpiece. Tungsten-carbide tipped burs designed for surgical use are ideal for cutting bone. Sharp new stainless steel burs are also adequate for the purpose, but they become blunt very quickly and should then be discarded. Blunt burs do not cut effectively but generate excessive heat at the bone surface.

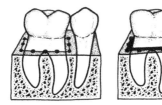

Figure 3.9. Removal of a block of bone by the 'postage stamp' method.

All burs must be cooled by plentiful irrigation with sterile saline delivered precisely to the interface of bur and bone. A rise in temperature of just 10 degrees is lethal to osteocytes and an uncooled bur cutting bone for only a few seconds will readily exceed this and burn the bone. A useful secondary effect of the cooling irrigation fluid is to wash away bone debris and blood from the operative field, thus helping to maintain clear visual access and preventing the bur blades from becoming clogged.

Bone removal can be adequately accomplished using a slow or mid-range speed handpiece designed for restorative dental procedures, provided that a suitable irrigant fluid can be delivered at a sufficient flow rate to cool the bur. However, air turbines that operate at high speed and spray a mixture of air and water under high pressure are inappropriate for surgical use as they may force air under the flap and into the tissues causing surgical emphysema.

Bone can be removed in one of two ways using a bur. The bone surface can simply be shaved down with a bur large enough to be effective (size number 8–12, round or fissure pattern), or else a block of bone is outlined using a smaller bur and the whole piece then dislodged (Figure 3.9).

Rosehead (round) burs   are versatile and efficient in that they can cut in any direction and have less of a tendency to clog with particles of bone than fissure burs. It is, however, more difficult to control the direction of lateral cuts using a round bur, and once the head of the bur is buried in bone, judgement of cutting depth is curtailed.

Fissure burs   cut neatly and precisely in a lateral direction but are less good than round burs at drilling penetrating holes. Because the cutting blades of a fissure bur cut a little less aggressively, the operator has a greater 'feel' through the instrument of what is being cut and this helps in distinguishing the difference in hardness between bone and dentine. This feature can be exploited in drilling away bone around a root surface as the bur preferentially cuts the bone and less readily penetrates the root. A medium sized fissure bur (number 6) is a good choice for removing bone in this way (the 'guttering' technique) thus making a space for a small elevator.

TOOTH REMOVAL

Making a point of application

Atlas said 'give me a lever and a secure fulcrum and I will move the world'. Without a fulcrum, or application point, elevators, like levers, are ineffective. Normally suitable points of application can be made by removing bone around the root as described above. The positioning of these points must take into account the shape of the roots and their possible direction of displacement (see section on use of elevators in Chapter 2). Sometimes it is necessary to make a more secure place for the elevator to engage the root by drilling a small notch in its side (Figure 3.10). The notch should be cut so as to leave the root dentine above it sufficiently well supported that it does not fracture with the force of elevation. Thus the notch is either cut well away from the edge of the root face or angled from it as shown in the diagram.

In the removal of multi-rooted teeth, usually the most difficult root to elevate is the *first* one. The space in the socket left by the extraction of the first root is then available to provide further and deeper application points for the remaining roots by breaking through the inter-radicular septa of bone with angled elevators, either Warwick–James', or where space permits, Cryer's. It follows from this principle that the best root to remove first in such a tooth is the one most accessible both for its own elevation and for the subsequent position of the application point(s) achieved.

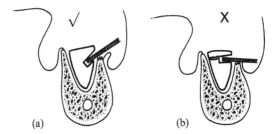

Figure 3.10. Cutting a notch in the root to provide a more secure grip for an elevator. (a) Correct depth and angulation of notch; (b) notch too close to root surface leading to fracture.

Tooth division

Dividing a tooth is indicated when the intact tooth is resisting displacement, yet the parts of the tooth – individual roots and crown – could be more easily removed after separation from each other. There are two common examples of this:

(a) Roots that are widely divergent with different paths of withdrawal; lower molars often show this pattern. Root division is most readily accomplished after sectioning the crown and then cutting between the roots with a fissure bur (number 6) starting at the bifurcation and moving coronally until the roots are separated. It is much easier to ensure that the roots are completely divided through the furcation by beginning at that point. Cutting down from the crown of the tooth, the bur may not locate the bifurcation and merely split off a part of one root, leaving the remainder of it still solidly joined. Once separated, the individual roots are displaced, each along its own path of withdrawal using a small elevator such as a number 1 Coupland's. (Figure 3.11).

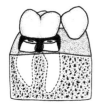

Figure 3.11. Division of the roots and sectioning of the crown.

(b) Impacted teeth where the path of withdrawal is blocked by the adjacent tooth in the arch. Lower second premolars demonstrate this problem if the tooth is trapped in insufficient space between the first premolar and first molar, with the crown wedged against one of these teeth and the root close to the other (Figure 3.12a, b, c). Sectioning the crown from the root with a fissure bur greatly facilitates the displacement of both, and minimizes the requirement for bone removal. It should also create enough space to permit removal of the crown in a buccal direction. Note that the angle of the bur is critical when sectioning a tooth for this purpose. It is possible to leave the crown still locked in position if the bur makes an oblique cut from above, and the coronal fragment is bigger lingually than buccally. Once the crown is removed, there should be sufficient room into which the root can be elevated.

Before dividing teeth, it is advisable to remove enough bone round the roots to provide suitable application points for elevators. It is much easier for the operator to see where bone removal is required with the tooth still intact, and it also simplifies sectioning the tooth at the correct angle if more of its root is visible. Surgical 'orientation' on the root tends to be lost if tooth division leaves the root fragment deeply buried in bone. Dental burs provide the most versatile and predictable method of tooth division and, with modern surgical drills,

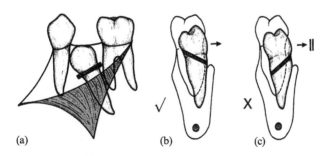

(a) (b) (c)

Figure 3.12. (a) Buccal view of impacted lower second premolar showing division of the crown from the root. (b) Cross-section through the alveolus – note the angle of the tooth division to permit removal of the crown. (c) Line of division angled incorrectly, blocking the removal of the crown in a buccal direction.

tooth structure is readily cut. An alternative method some-times preferred by experienced operators is to split the tooth with an *osteotome*, an instrument like a chisel but with a bevel on both sides of its cutting tip. Although this technique is quicker than the bur, it has several disadvantages:

- No space is created for instrumentation or movement between the separated fragments.
- The tooth may not split along the intended line.
- The technique is not safe in inexperienced hands (see Chapter 5).

Not all teeth are suitable to be divided, and in some cases sectioning the crown can make removal of the root even more difficult. This is true of teeth where the only safe, solid and accessible point of application for an elevator, or the best position to grasp the tooth with forceps, is by its crown. Disto-angularly inclined lower third molars and canines or second premolars in the palate often demonstrate this conundrum. Careful further removal of bone around the root, after assessing the cause of the obstruction and prior to re-attempting displacement of the intact tooth, is normally the best policy.

Elevation of roots

The principles of root elevation following bone removal are identical to those described in Chapter 2. However, removing bone provides the opportunity to gain optimal application points for elevation and to clear the path of exit of the root. The effectiveness of elevation is thereby substantially enhanced. In some situations it may also be possible, and indeed preferable, to reach a root using fine-bladed forceps. If, even after removing bone, a root fragment is resistant to elevation or is difficult to reach effectively with elevators, then a decision must be taken about whether to leave the remaining root in situ. In general it is better to leave a small piece of root behind than to risk damage to nearby structures during heroic attempts to remove it. Most root fragments left in this way do not cause any complication unless the remnant is large and prevents the socket from healing, or the root is infected. Non-vital roots and roots that have been dislodged during the extraction attempt, only to become stuck fast elsewhere in the socket, should ideally be removed as they may be a nidus for infection.

FOLLOWING TOOTH REMOVAL

Debridement of the socket

Once the tooth has been successfully removed, the socket should be cleaned and checked for pieces of debris that could impede healing. Thorough aspiration using vacuum suction and a fine surgical sucker tip allows close inspection of the wound and may remove small loose pieces of bone, tooth or filling material. Larger fragments are best retrieved with fine curved artery forceps. Irrigation with sterile saline is helpful in providing a clear view and flushing out small particles safely from the depths of the socket. Gentle curettage of the bony socket walls with the spoon end of a Mitchell's trimmer removes any remnants of adherent infected granulation tissue from the periodontium. However, misguidedly over-enthusiastic prodding with instruments in deep recesses of the wound could result in damage to delicate nearby structures such as the inferior dental nerve or the thin bone plate of the antral floor.

Any unwanted bony prominences or sharp edges around the socket should be reduced using the rongeur bone nibblers or an acrylic bur in a handpiece run at slow speed. The wound is now ready for closure.

Suturing

The main purposes of suturing are as follows:

- To replace and secure the mucoperiosteal flap in its former position.

- To limit the size of the wound and therefore restrict subsequent contamination with food debris.
- To assist in controlling haemorrhage.
- To retain the position of a flap advanced over the opening of a socket (i.e. in the repair of an oro–antral communication – see Chapter 5).

Suture materials are either absorbable (they are broken down by enzymatic degradation in the tissues) or non-absorbable, in which case they usually need to be removed after 7–10 days. The thread may be formed of a single thick filament, that tends to have springy 'elastic memory' which makes the stitch more difficult to tie, or many thin filaments braided together to make a material that is easier to use and holds knots better.

Those most commonly used in oral surgical procedures are:

- Black silk – a non-absorbable braided natural material; probably the most widely used because it handles so well.
- Vicryl (Ethicon) – a slowly absorbable braided synthetic thread with handling characteristics close to silk.
- Catgut – an absorbable mono-filament collagenous material extracted from the intestines of sheep.

The most appropriate gauge (thickness) for each of the above suture materials is 3/0.

Needles for suturing vary in size, curvature, and profile of their cutting point. The most versatile needle for use in repositioning mucoperiosteal flaps has a slim body with a length from 19 to 22 mm, a curvature of 3/8ths of the circumference of a circle, and a sharp triangular shaped profile at its point. Such a needle is called 'cutting', or 'reverse cutting' according to the orientation of the triangular cross-section. These characteristics enable the needle to fit through the interdental spaces, to pass easily through the soft tissues in a curved arc, and still be retrieved even in the most awkward distal parts of the mouth. All sutures suitable for oral surgery have the needle attached to one end of the thread so that the join passes atraumatically through the tissues; hence the name 'atraumatic' needle (as opposed to a needle with an eye in its tail through which the thread was passed).

The body of the needle (not the sharp cutting end or the tail) is grasped in the jaws of *needle holders* near their tips and at an angle to suit the direction of access to the operative site (Figure 3.13).

It is simplest to use a needle holder about 7 inches in length with ratchet gripped handles. The mobile tissue of the flap should be stabilized by using toothed tissue forceps to hold the flap near, but not directly at, its free edge. The rat-toothed beaks enable the soft tissue to be held without slipping off the flap or crushing its margin (Figure 3.14a, b).

Suturing techniques

Three basic patterns of stitches are commonly used in the mouth:

- Interrupted sutures are individually tied and have a single 'bite' of tissue on each side of the incision to approximate the edges (Figure 3.15a). They are the most useful and versatile type of stitch.
- Mattress sutures have a double 'bite' of tissue on each side of the soft tissues so that when tightened, the suture everts the approximated wound margins and provides more secure closure, particularly if the soft tissues are friable and liable to tear. The two bites of tissue may be arranged horizontally or vertically (Figure 3.15b, c).
- Continuous sutures are useful when a longer length of flap is to be repositioned following the extraction of several adjacent teeth. The suture runs without interruption from one end of the wound to the other and because it is only tied at each end it is quick to place. After each pair of bites in opposite sides of the wound, the needle is passed under the free loop of thread, so 'locking' the suture continually along its length. This is the equivalent of a blanket stitch in needlework (Figure 3.15d).

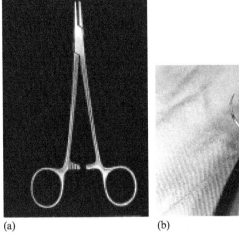
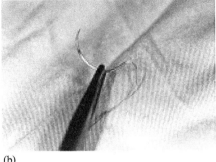

(a)   (b)

Figure 3.13. (a) Needle holder with ratchet handles. (b) Body of a curved cutting needle held correctly at the tip of the needle holder.

The following key principles of technique apply to each of the suture patterns listed above:

- The needle should take a secure bite of the soft tissues about 3 mm from their free edge. Any closer and the stitch may tear out, whilst bigger bites may lead to less accurate replacement of the flap margins or cause the tissues to fold up under the stitch as it is tightened.
- In general it is better to suture from the free tissue of the flap towards the fixed tissues opposite.
- The needle should be passed through the tissues one side of the wound at a time with a separate pass for the second side. This ensures optimal angulation and needle position for each bite of the tissue without any undue tension on the tissues of the flap.
- The needle is curved and must be advanced through the tissue on a curved track. Any attempt to push the needle straight through may result in it cutting out of the flap sideways (remember the needle has sharp cutting edges, not merely a sharpened tip).
- In places in the mouth where access is awkward, such as the buccal sulcus in the third molar area, it can be

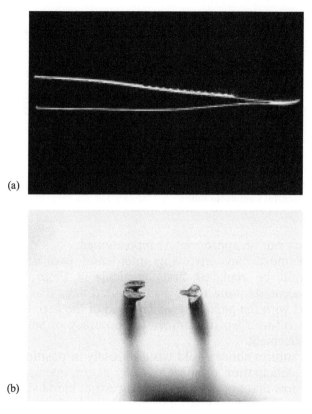

(a)

(b)

Figure 3.14. (a) Rat-toothed tissue forceps with (b) detail of the tissue-holding teeth.

difficult to retrieve the needle from the tissues. It is usually easy to put the needle into the desired place, but it may be extremely hard to get the needle to turn along its curved path far enough for the tip to re-emerge from the depths of the concavity that is the back of the mouth. A little forethought when aligning the needle on entering the tissues may help to ensure there is an accessible exit route.

- Once the suture thread is placed and before tying the knot, the effectiveness of the stitch can be checked by gently pulling the flap with the suture and approximating the wound margins. If the result is unsatisfactory the

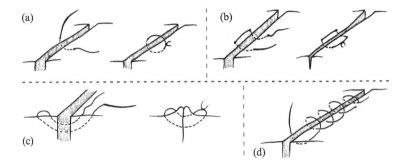

Figure 3.15. (a) Interrupted suture. (b) Horizontal mattress suture. (c) Vertical mattress suture. (d) Continuous suture.

stitch can be appropriately repositioned.

- For most flaps involving interdental papillae, these should be replaced first, particularly those around adjacent standing teeth. In two-sided flaps it is best to start with the papilla at the free end of the flap; this first key suture then determines the accuracy of soft tissue replacement.
- All sutures should hold tissues loosely in position, with the anticipation of some swelling at the operative site. Sutures that are too tight merely restrict blood supply to the margins of the flap and may delay healing.
- The knots should be placed to one side of the wound rather than directly over it.

Tying the knot

Tying knots in the mouth is easiest using the needle holder rather than the fingers. Figure 3.16 shows the sequence of steps necessary. Note that each component of the knot is called a 'throw'. These may be single or double according to how many times the thread is wound around the needle holder. Single throws slide more easily from the needle holder but may slip more readily when in position before a second, or 'locking throw', can be placed. Practice using a piece of felt or similar material on a board is strongly recommended before getting yourself tied up in knots in a patient's mouth.

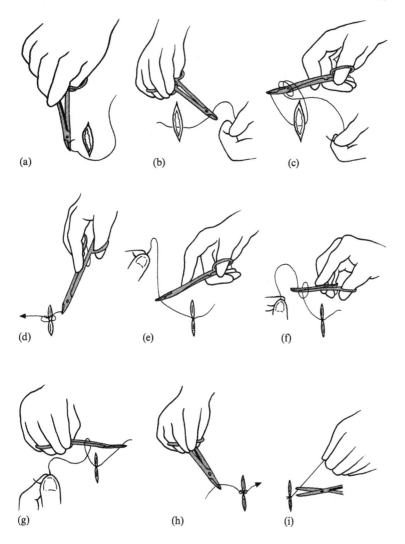

Figure 3.16. Tying a surgical knot using a needle holder. (b) The thread is wound twice around the needle holder in a 'forwards' direction. (c) The first throw has a double loop that draws the margins of the wound together when tightened. (f) The second throw is a single loop around the needle holder in the opposite direction to the first; it locks the knot in position.

Post-operative care

The aftercare of trans-alveolar extractions is broadly similar to that described in Chapter 2 for intra-alveolar procedures with the following additional considerations.

(a) Antibiotic therapy. When any significant amount of bone is removed, it may be appropriate to prescribe a 3–5 day course of antibiotic therapy to reduce the risk of post-operative wound infection. Metronidazole 200 mg tds or penicillin V 250 mg qds are logical choices for this purpose, provided the patient has no history of adverse reaction to the drug selected. Although most dental surgeons, including the author, would adhere to this recommendation in their practice, the topic remains a source of controversy with conflicting evidence in the literature about the justification of giving antibiotics routinely to all such patients for the benefit of the few prevented from developing infections. It must be realized, however, that spreading oro-facial infections from the jaws carry a significant morbidity and can, albeit rarely, be lethal. There is no dissent from the view that immuno-compromised patients should be given antibiotics prophylactically.

(b) Suture removal. When non-absorbable sutures have been placed they should be removed, normally after about 7 days. In some cases where absorbable sutures were used, they are still present after this time and the patient may find it preferable to have them removed if they are irritating the tongue. Sutures placed to control haemorrhage can be removed after 48 hours, whilst those used to repair oro–antral communications are left in situ for 10 days.

(c) Post-surgical review. It is not always necessary to see every patient for a post-operative review; however there should be the facility for any patients experiencing post-operative problems to seek advice or to be seen without undue delay.

Examples of trans-alveolar tooth removal

Maxillary first permanent molar with widely splayed roots

Pre-operative radiographic assessment of this tooth reveals that the roots are widely divergent and thus have conflicting paths of withdrawal (Figure 3.17). Successful forceps extraction of the tooth would depend on the elasticity of the bone as the socket must be dilated considerably to allow the passage of the roots without fracture of either bone or tooth. This may be possible in the young patient, but less likely if the bone is unyielding. Therefore a decision taken at the outset to tackle this tooth by a trans-alveolar method transforms a difficult and potentially traumatic extraction with an uncertain outcome into a comparatively straightforward and predictable surgical procedure. Figure 3.18 shows the key stages.

1. A two-sided flap offers adequate access (Figure 3.18b).
2. Bone removal with a bur to expose the furcation of the two buccal roots (Figure 3.18c).
3. The buccal roots are sectioned *close to* the furcation with a fissure bur. The palatal root is still attached to the crown of the tooth (Figure 3.18d, e).
4. The crown is carefully extracted along with the palatal root using upper molar forceps. Gentle buccal movement is recommended to avoid breaking the root (Figure 3.18e).
5. The two buccal roots are elevated separately.
6. After debridement of the socket, the flap is sutured. The first stitch repositions the papilla at the free end of the flap, next the relieving incision is sutured and lastly a stitch across the middle of the socket minimizes the gape of the wound. Note that it is not possible to close the mouth of the socket, and any attempt to do so will merely drag the flap out of position and cause the relieving incision to gape open. Placement of a stitch across the socket before the corner of the flap is secured also produces the same unwanted effect (Figure 3.18f).

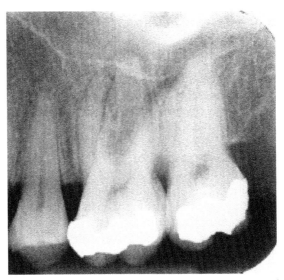

Figure 3.17. Radiograph of an upper first molar with splayed roots.

Mandibular first permanent molar

Bone in the posterior part of the mandibular alveolus is often dense and unyielding. When the roots of a molar tooth curve towards each other, they effectively 'grasp' the bone between them which would then prevent their removal unless either root or bone is fractured. Figure 3.19 shows the radiograph of a root-treated (and therefore brittle) lower first molar in a man aged 50 with a history of difficult extractions. Attempted forceps extraction is likely to result in the fracture of this tooth at or below bone level, leaving the roots buried inaccessibly in the dense bone. A planned surgical approach in the following way offers a more controllable procedure with a more predictable outcome:

1. A two-sided flap is cut with the relieving incision kept well away from the mental nerve as it emerges from the mental foramen located just below and between the apices of the premolar teeth (Figure 3.20a).
2. Bone is removed with a bur, first outlining the area for

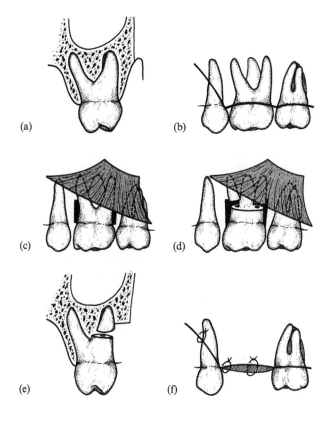

(a)

(b)

(c)

(d)

(e)

(f)

Figure 3.18. Diagrams showing stages (described in the text) of the surgical removal of the tooth in Figure 3.17.

resection using the 'postage stamp' method, and then cutting the block of bone free and so exposing the bifurcation and a few millimetres of the roots. This technique is much quicker than laboriously shaving down through thick dense mandibular cortical bone (Figure 3.20b).

3. The crown is sectioned from the roots which are then separated from each other with a bur. Note that the coronal portions of the roots have been left showing above bone level to expedite their subsequent elevation (Figure 3.20c).

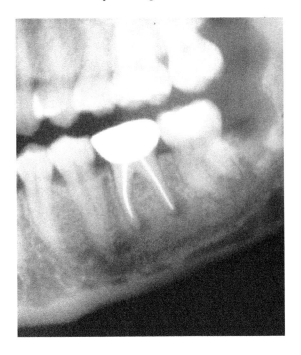

Figure 3.19. Radiograph of a brittle non-vital mandibular first molar in dense bone.

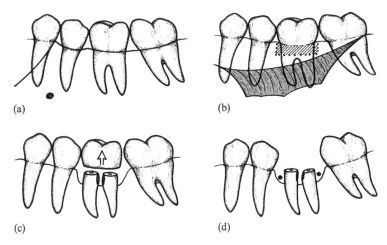

(a)   (b)

(c)   (d)

Figure 3.20. Diagrams showing stages (described in the text) of the surgical removal of the tooth in Figure 3.19.

4. The roots can now be elevated along their different paths of withdrawal, the mesial root curving distally from a mesial point of application, and the distal root in the opposite direction (Figure 3.20d).
5. After cleaning the wound, the flap is sutured in the manner described above for the upper molar extraction.

Chapter 4

Extractions under general anaesthesia

The vast majority of dental extractions are carried out under local anaesthesia. However, there remains a small proportion of teeth that are more appropriately removed under general anaesthesia. Pre-operative assessment of the patient, involving the medical history, the anticipated level of co-operation and the complexity of the surgical task in hand, is mandatory before a logical choice of anaesthetic technique can be made. The indications and contraindications for general anaesthesia with regard to the patient's medical history are set out in Chapter 1.

Assessment for general anaesthesia

General anaesthetics used to be employed much more commonly for dental extractions, and even dental clearances in 'the chair' using inhalational anaesthesia without endotracheal intubation were routine. Over the past two or three decades changing attitudes to general anaesthesia, in particular the safety aspect, have led to a series of modifications to recommended practice for the administration of general anaesthesia that have restricted its use in dental surgery. The Poswillo report published in 1990 on general anaesthesia in dentistry, as well as modified regulations introduced by the General Dental Council (GDC) in 1998, give clear guidance towards realization of the small but significant risk of general anaesthesia and the desirability of using local anaesthesia on safety grounds for dental extractions when possible. Poswillo stated that 'general anaesthesia for dental purposes should continue to be available in dental surgeries and clinics where this is clinically justified', and that 'the same standards of monitoring and personnel, necessary for patient safety, shall apply wherever general anaesthetics are administered'. The availability of effective alternative techniques such as intravenous or inhalational sedation has also helped to enhance patient acceptance of local anaesthetics for dental surgery. The GDC, in its publication 'Maintaining Standards', makes the following statement: 'General anaesthesia is a procedure which is never without risk. In assessing the needs of an individual patient, due regard should be given to all aspects of behavioural management and anxiety control before deciding to prescribe or to proceed with treatment under general anaesthesia'. The document goes on to require that dentists observe the following before referring patients for general anaesthesia:

- Full medical history must be taken.
- Risks of general anaesthesia to be explained to the patient as well as the alternative methods of pain control.
- Justification for the use of general anaesthesia and details of relevant medical or dental history to be included in the referral letter.
- Written consent signed by the patient.
- Clear pre- and post-operative instructions given to the patient in written form.

The person administering the general anaesthesia must be recognized as a specialist in anaesthesia by the General Medical Council and have available for assistance an individual specifically trained and experienced in the necessary skills to assist in monitoring the patient's condition and in any emergency. There must also be full patient monitoring and resuscitation equipment available along with a protocol for the provision of advanced life support including arrangements for immediate transfer of a patient to a critical care facility.

Sedation administered either by the intravenous route using a single drug such as midazolam, or by inhalation (nitrous oxide/oxygen relative analgesia), is a useful practical alternative to general anaesthesia for the anxious patient. The GDC regulations for sedation (as of 1998) require:

- The dentist administering the sedation must have experience and postgraduate training but may act as operator and sedationist provided a second appropriately trained person is present throughout who is capable of monitoring the clinical condition of the patient and of assisting in the case of an emergency.
- Full medical history taken.
- Written pre- and post-operative instructions.
- Standards of monitoring recommended in the guidelines of the Resuscitation Council are followed.
- Drugs for resuscitation are available.
- The patient has an escort.
- Written consent must be obtained.

Oral sedation with small doses of diazepam or temazepam given 1–2 hours pre-operatively can be helpful to the nervous patient. An escort is required for such occasions but no additional safety procedures or regulations apply to this technique.

Preparation of the patient for general anaesthesia

(a) Escort.   Most patients attending for dental extractions under general anaesthesia will be treated as a day case. They are required to be accompanied by a responsible adult who will escort them home preferably by car or taxi, but in some circumstances public transport may be appropriate.

(b) Nil by mouth.   The patient should have nothing to eat or drink for 6 hours before the anaesthetic. A few sips of water to facilitate the swallowing of essential medication may be permitted.

(c) Clothing.   Many hospital day case units provide theatre gowns for patients to wear. If their own clothing is to be retained, shoes should be removed and all tight garments especially belts and collars loosened.

(d) Bladder.   All patients should be encouraged to empty

their bladder before the induction of anaesthesia to avoid embarrassing mishaps due to loss of sphincter control.

(e) Chaperone. Female patients should ideally be chaperoned by a female member of staff.

(f) Preparation of the mouth. Removable prostheses must be removed to ensure a clear airway. Note should be taken of any crowns or bridges especially on anterior teeth and the anaesthetist informed. The upper incisors are particularly vulnerable to pressure from the laryngoscope.

Alteration of extraction technique for general anaesthesia

Access

When under anaesthesia, patients are co-operative but passively so. A prop is required to maintain the mouth open and retraction of the tongue and cheeks may be needed as shown in Figure 4.1c. Adequate access is important to facilitate safe operating, but a balance must be found between the need to open the mouth widely and the possibility of overstretching the temporomandibular joints and causing them to dislocate. Note that a smaller prop pushed well back in the mouth gives the same opening as a larger one placed further forwards, but takes up less of the operating space.

Positioning of the patient and operator

In virtually all cases the patient will be supine, as this is the preferred safe position for general anaesthesia. The operator should adopt an approach to the mouth using the guidelines set out in Chapter 2. In general, a right-handed surgeon will perform forceps extractions of teeth in the upper and lower right, as well as the upper left quadrants, from the right side of the chair or operating table, and teeth in the lower left quadrant from the left side. However, the ambidextrous surgeon can carry out extractions in any part of the mouth from the head of the table (if lower forceps are used for the upper teeth).

Airway protection

The operating environment in the mouth must be sealed off in some way from the pharynx to prevent blood, saliva and pieces of tooth or dental filling from falling back over the tongue with the danger of entering the trachea. The most common site for such a foreign body to lodge is the right main bronchus, and the likely result is a lung abscess. Protection of the airway can be achieved in several ways.

1. Anaesthesia using a nasal mask and an oral pack.   A 6 cm width of gamgee gauze cut to a length of about 30 cm is placed to the side of the tongue in a double fold extending from the lingual sulcus up to the palate on the side of the extraction. The tail of the pack is also brought around the last standing upper and lower teeth in the retromolar area to reach the buccal vestibule. In this way any debris from the extraction will either be adsorbed or lodged in the pack. The technique of positioning such a pack is as follows (Figure 4.1). A double fold of gamgee gauze is held with the 'tail' of the pack just beyond two fingertips (Figure 4.1a). A sweeping motion retracts the tongue sideways (do NOT push it back – otherwise the airway will be obstructed) and places the lower part of the pack in the lingual sulcus. The tail end of the pack falls around the retromolar region into the cheek (Figure 4.1b, c).

It must be understood that an oral pack can only absorb so much blood, and if the extraction is prolonged or the haemorrhage is significant then the pack may become soaked despite diligent efforts with the sucker. Once saturated, the pack will then leak fluid back towards an unprotected airway. Therefore the mouth pack method is only suitable for predictably short, simple extraction procedures, e.g. with one or two teeth, preferably on the same side of the mouth. The time available for operating is necessarily limited (5–10 minutes at most) when the mouth pack is the sole form of airway protection. The additional difficulty with this method is that whilst the operating area of the mouth has to be packed off, the airway from the nasopharynx over the back of the tongue must remain patent with the tongue and lower jaw

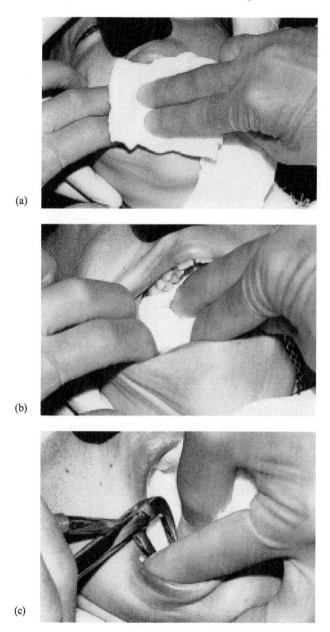

(a)

(b)

(c)

Figure 4.1. Stages in the placement of an oral pack to protect the airway from debris from the mouth and to absorb blood.

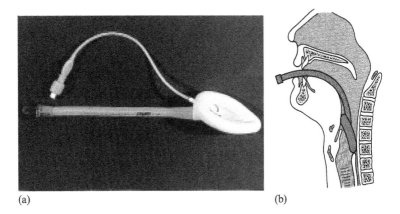

(a)   (b)

Figure 4.2. (a) Laryngeal mask with flexible armoured (unsquashable) tube.
(b) Diagram of a laryngeal mask in position seen in the sagittal plane.

pulled forwards to ensure this. The operator needs to understand the importance of supporting the jaw with the left hand to maintain the airway whilst the anaesthetist pursues the same ends by pushing the angles of the mandible forwards from behind as well as holding the nasal mask in position. To be successful the operator and anaesthetist must work closely as a team with each member performing his own task and understanding the role of the other. The anaesthetist however remains in overall charge of the airway and in this regard is the boss. In case of airway difficulty, the anaesthetist dictates the strategy and the operation may need to be suspended whilst the airway is re-established either via the nasal mask or by inserting a laryngeal mask or else passing an endotracheal tube.

2. The laryngeal mask   enables the airway to be sealed off from the mouth by covering the laryngeal inlet with an inflatable diaphragm connected to an oral airway tube (Figure 4.2a, b). This affords excellent airway protection in itself, but also allows a gauze throat pack to be placed over the back of the tongue into the oropharynx thus providing a second line of defence. Placement of a laryngeal mask does not require the patient to be paralysed or deeply anaesthe-

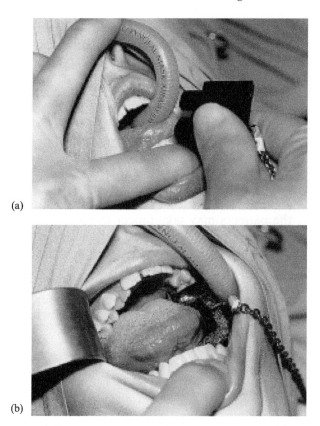

(a)

(b)

Figure 4.3. (a), (b) Positioning of the laryngeal mask tube behind the mouth prop.

tized as nothing is inserted through the larynx past the vocal cords (as is the case with endotracheal tubes).

Once the laryngeal mask is in position the extraction procedure can go ahead safely without the time constraints that apply with a mouth pack alone. The only disadvantage of the laryngeal mask is the oral tube which can get in the way of some intra-oral procedures, but this restriction of access is minimized by armoured (unsquashable) tubes that can be bent around behind the prop on the contralateral side of the mouth (Figure 4.3a, b).

3. An endotracheal tube may be passed through the nose thus avoiding any obstruction to the operator in the mouth. The tip of the tube enters the trachea via the larynx and must therefore pass the vocal cords. In order to overcome the extremely powerful cough reflex provoked by touching the cords, the patient must either be deeply unconscious or paralysed with a muscle relaxant drug. Endotracheal anaesthesia is therefore more appropriate for prolonged or difficult surgical procedures rather than simple extractions, or may be preferred where access to an awkward part of the mouth would be obstructed by the oral tube of a laryngeal mask. The operating conditions provided by a nasal tube are optimal. However, the patients may take longer to recover from this type of anaesthesia before being fit for discharge with their escort, and they often complain of a sore throat post-operatively following the intubation.

If the appropriate type of anaesthetic has been chosen, there should be ample time to complete any extraction procedure. The days of 'smash and grab' anaesthetics have passed.

Modifications of extraction technique for general anaesthesia

- Care should be taken with soft tissues that may fall passively into harm's way in the unconscious patient. The cheeks, lips or tongue can be trapped by the forceps or crushed against nearby teeth.
- In cases of multiple extractions, remove roots and difficult teeth first.
- Stabilize the jaw with the left (non-extracting) hand to avoid excessive force being transmitted to the temporo-mandibular joints when the jaw muscles are relaxed and offer no support.
- Remove any debris including bits of tooth or filling immediately they become loose to prevent their loss into the pharynx or beyond.
- Check all areas of the mouth for pieces of debris *before* removing the pack.
- Check the occlusion of the teeth at the end of the

procedure to ensure the jaw has not been dislocated.
- Suction is essential at all times. A back-up apparatus should be available in case of equipment failure.
- Full surgical instrumentation should be available for use if needed, so that no surgical task is left unnecessarily unfinished.

Chapter 5
Complications of tooth extraction

No surgical procedure is guaranteed to be free of complications and tooth extraction is no exception. Whilst the risk of
certain adverse events can be minimized with forethought at
the assessment stage and careful execution of the surgery,
some of the problems that arise are totally unpredictable.

Complications of tooth extraction are many and varied.
They may present immediately at the time of surgery or
become manifest at different intervals post-operatively. Most
problems occur locally in the mouth, but others are systemic
events.

LOCAL COMPLICATIONS

Immediate

- Failure of local anaesthesia.
- Failure to move the tooth.
- Fracture of the tooth or root being extracted.
- Fracture of the alveolus (including maxillary tuberosity).
- Oro–antral communication.
- Displacement of the tooth or a root into the tissues.
- Loss of a tooth or part of a tooth into the pharynx and
  thence to the lung or stomach.
- Fracture or subluxation of an adjacent tooth.
- Collateral damage to surrounding soft tissues.
- Thermal injury.
- Haemorrhage.
- Dislocation of the temporomandibular joint.
- Fracture of the mandible.
- Damage to branches of the trigeminal nerve.

Delayed

- Excessive pain, swelling and trismus.
- Haemorrhage.
- Localized osteitis (dry socket).
- Acute osteomyelitis.
- Infection of soft tissues.
- Oro–antral fistula.
- Failure of the socket to heal.
- Nerve damage.

Late

- Chronic osteomyelitis.
- Osteoradionecrosis.
- Nerve damage.
- Chronic pain.

SYSTEMIC COMPLICATIONS

Immediate

- Faint (vaso-vagal attack).
- Hypoglycaemia.
- Panic attack/hyperventilation.
- Convulsions/fits.
- Myocardial infarction.
- Addisonian crisis.
- Respiratory obstruction.

Late

- Infective endocarditis.
- Transmissible viral infections, e.g. hepatitis.

DEALING WITH LOCAL COMPLICATIONS

Failure of local anaesthesia is usually the result of either inaccurate placement of the anaesthetic solution, too small a dosage, or not waiting long enough for the anaesthesia to develop before commencing surgery. Both patient and operator need to know that the anaesthetic is working satisfactorily before the extraction can proceed with the comfort and confidence of both parties. A simple test of adequate numbness is to push a blunt probe firmly into the gingival crevice around the tooth for extraction. Whilst the patient will feel the transmitted pressure from the probe there should be no sensation of sharpness or pain. An additional precaution is to tap the tooth with a mirror handle as occasionally a tooth that is periostitic, and therefore would be painful to extract, is not detected using the probe test. If anaesthesia cannot be secured by using conventional techniques of infiltration or regional block, intraligamental, intraosseous or intrapulpal injections may be indicated, provided that the cause of the failure is not local infection around the tooth. Local anaesthetic should not be injected into infected tissues because of the risk of spreading the infection.

Failure to move the tooth. If the tooth does not yield to reasonable displacing forces applied with forceps or elevators, this normally indicates that either the bone texture is dense and inelastic, or that the root shape is obstructing its path of withdrawal. To persevere with forceps using ever greater force is likely to result in fracture of the tooth or exhaustion of both the operator and the patient. The cause of the obstruction should be sought, taking a radiograph (if a satisfactory film showing *the whole* of the root is not already available) before proceeding to lift a mucoperiosteal flap and remove bone and/or divide the tooth as indicated (see Chapter 3).

Fracture of the tooth. The *causes* of crown or root fracture are:

- Excessive force applied to the tooth.
- A tooth weakened by caries or large restorations.
- Inappropriate application of force resulting from failure

to grasp enough of the root mass or using forceps with blades too wide to make two point contact on the root (see Chapter 2).

- Haste due to impatience or frustration.
- Unfavourable root anatomy.

Tooth fracture is an inconvenience, but need not be a disaster, and it happens to even the most experienced exodontists! The key to managing this potential problem is to *reassess* the situation and decide whether to proceed, or abort the extraction attempt and refer the patient for oral surgical advice. Inspection of the fractured tooth shows the likely size and position of the retained root. If there is no pre-operative radiograph that shows the whole of the root structure then one should be taken at this stage. When only the crown has been removed, it may be possible to reapply root forceps, but this is unlikely to be productive unless there is a reasonable amount of root accessible above alveolar bone level, and the root has already shown signs of loosening. When the root itself has fractured, retrieval of the retained portion normally requires a surgical approach. The operator must assess whether this surgical task is feasible given the co-operation of the patient, the facilities available and his or her level of experience.

Ideally all roots should be removed but some apical fragments may be difficult or hazardous to pursue because of the proximity of the inferior dental nerve or the antral floor. Such small apices are best left in situ and rarely cause symptoms. In general, a root fragment of a vital tooth, less than 5 mm in length, can normally be safely left in the jaws of healthy patients. Larger root fragments and those with necrotic pulps or periapical radiolucent areas should be removed, unless the risk of so doing outweighs the potential gain. In patients who are immunocompromised or at risk of infective endocarditis, all potential causes of infection should be removed whenever possible. If it is decided that the root can be safely retained, then the patient must be informed of this eventuality along with a suitable explanation, and both the retention of the root apex and the information given to the patient should be recorded in the clinical notes.

When the retrieval of the root is deemed to be advisable but is beyond the capability of the operator, then the procedure should be stopped, any accessible exposed vital pulp tissue removed, the wound closed with sutures (if appropriate) and suitable medication (analgesics and antibiotics) prescribed. A full explanation should be given to the patient who is then referred, preferably by telephone or fax, for further management by an oral surgeon.

Fracture of the alveolus is a common occurrence during tooth extraction; small pieces of alveolar bone are often adherent to a root and are removed with it. Occasionally a larger fragment of bone is fractured as the tooth is loosened and this too may have to be removed if the tooth cannot be separated from it. In this case the soft tissue should be dissected from the loose bone using an instrument such as a Mitchell's trimmer, to avoid tearing the gingiva as the tooth and bone fragment are delivered. It is sometimes possible to detach the bone fragment from the tooth with a fine fissure bur or a Coupland's chisel, and provided the loose bone has secure attachment to soft tissue (and therefore a sound blood supply), it can be safely retained.

Fracture of the maxillary tuberosity is a particular type of alveolar fracture which may be predisposed by:

- the presence of a large antrum that weakens the maxillary alveolus
- a large or splayed root mass of the upper second or third molar
- fusion of an unerupted third molar to the root of the second molar (see Figure 1.17c).

Small fragments of tuberosity fractured in this way normally need to be removed. This is achieved by raising a buccal flap large enough to permit a view of the fractured portion of tuberosity adherent to the tooth, and then dissecting the bone free from any remaining soft tissue. The tooth and the bone fragment are then removed together. If a large segment of alveolar bone is seen to move with the tooth, it may be advisable to abandon the extraction, give the patient a course of antibiotics and analgesics, then wait for 8–10 weeks for the fracture to heal before the tooth is removed by a surgical approach. Frequently the fracture includes that part of the bone forming the floor of the antrum and therefore a potential communication may have been created between the oral cavity and the nasal sinus. This requires special management as set out below.

Oro–antral communication. The root apices of the maxillary cheek teeth are closely related to the antral floor. With increasing age the nasal sinuses slowly enlarge so that the tooth roots often appear in a two-dimensional radiographic view to be protruding into the antral cavity (Figure 5.1). In three dimensions the thin bone of the antral floor undulates as it is draped over the angular contours of the root ends, and may be very thin or even show defects so that the root apices make contact with the antral lining (Figure 5.2). Appreciation of this anatomical relationship is important when removing any upper molar or premolar, but is particularly so in the elderly patient, where the bony barrier between tooth and sinus is thin and brittle. As the tooth is manipulated in the forceps, there is a risk that the bone of the antral floor, which may be adherent to the roots, will fracture and be removed with the tooth, so leaving a defect and creating a communication from the mouth to the antrum via the socket. This event may be immediately apparent on inspection of the extracted tooth if the bony fragment of the antral floor, with its characteristic smooth surface, is attached to the root apices (Figure 5.3). If a large defect has been created it may be possible to see the hole into the antrum at the base of the socket (Figure 5.4). If a communication is suspected but not identified by visual inspection of the socket or the tooth, the next step is to employ the nose blowing test. The patient should be instructed to blow *gently* through the nose against pinched nostrils to increase the intra-nasal pressure so that any patent defect will be disclosed by the passage of air into the socket. The air may produce bubbles with the blood in the socket, or if the socket is empty, a fine wisp of cotton wool held over the extraction site will be deflected by the stream of air. It is essential that only gentle pressure of air is used to

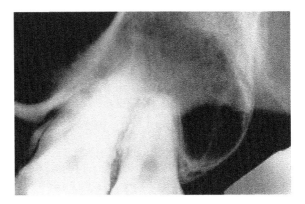

Figure 5.1. Upper molar roots apparently 'protruding' into the antrum when seen on a periapical radiograph.

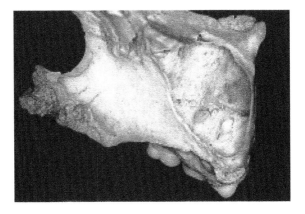

Figure 5.2. View inside the antral cavity in a disarticulated maxilla showing the root apices of the molar teeth visible through defects in the bone of the antral floor.

identify a communication; over-enthusiastic blowing may actually produce a breach of the antral soft tissue lining if this is left unsupported by a fracture of the bony antral wall. Similarly instruments such as sucker tips or probes should not be pushed up into the socket in an attempt to find a defect into the antrum as this manoeuvre could create a communication where none existed.

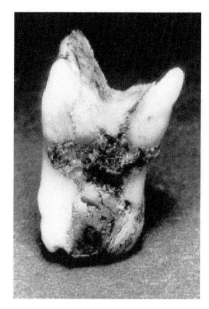

Figure 5.3. Extracted upper molar with a piece of the bony antral floor adherent to its roots.

Oro–antral communications are not normally predictable pre-operatively, but there are some features that may predispose to this complication:

- Large antral cavity extending between or around the roots of the teeth (Figure 5.1; see also Figure 1.13).
- A lone-standing tooth in an atrophic maxillary alveolus (see Figure 1.16).
- Molar teeth with large splayed roots close to the antral floor.
- Resistant third molars that threaten fracture of the maxillary tuberosity (see above).
- A history of antral involvement at previous extractions.

The ideal way to manage an oro–antral communication is to close it immediately before there is passage of infected material through the defect which may cause sinusitis. A three-sided buccal mucoperiosteal flap is raised and advanced over the open socket following release of the periosteum at the base of the flap well beyond the reflection of the sulcus. Once the unyielding periosteal layer is incised, there should be

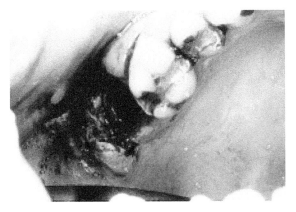

Figure 5.4. Inspection of the socket reveals a large defect through to the antrum.

sufficient mobility of the flap to reach the palatal side of the socket where it is secured with vertical mattress sutures (Figure 5.5a–e). Closure can be assisted by reducing the height of the socket walls. Post-operatively, a full explanation of events should be given to the patient and this is recorded in the notes with the operative details. The patient should also be advised to follow the instructions set out below; these measures are often referred to collectively as the 'antral regimen'.

- Avoid blowing the nose for 10–14 days (lest the repaired communication is breached).
- A broad spectrum antibiotic should be taken for 7 days to prevent sinus infection.
- Regular use of nasal inhalations of steam (usually with a camphorated medicament added) *or* nasal drops of ephedrine. Either of these measures is effective in helping to soften and clear mucus from the nose – the patient may be permitted to sniff or wipe, but not to blow!

If immediate surgical closure of the socket responsible for the oro–antral communication is not possible then the patient should be referred as soon as is practicable for management by an oral surgeon. The 'antral regimen' described above should in any case be started immediately. Once the

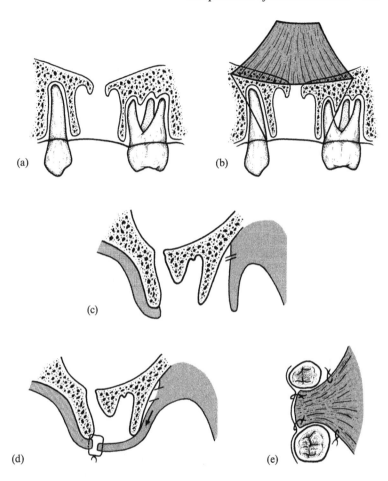

Figure 5.5. (a) Buccal view of upper first molar socket with an oro–antral communication. (b) Three-sided flap cut and raised well beyond the reflection of the buccal sulcus. (c) Cross-sectional view showing the site of the relieving incision through periosteum well above the reflection of the sulcus. (d) Advancement of the flap across the socket. (e) The flap sutured in position covering the socket.

communication between the mouth and the antrum becomes epithelialized, a tract called an oro–antral fistula is established and then requires formal surgical closure.

Displacement of a root into the antrum can occur following fracture of a maxillary molar or premolar and ineffective attempts to retrieve the retained palatal root. A large antral cavity close to the root apices is a predisposing factor, but the incidence of this complication could be reduced if the following basic rules were observed.

- Do not apply forceps to a root below the antrum unless there is sufficient exposure of the root to allow the blades to grasp the root securely under direct vision.
- Be content to leave the apical third of maxillary molar palatal roots, unless there is an overriding indication for their removal.

Never attempt to retrieve a root below the antrum by passing an instrument *up* into the tooth socket. Rather raise a buccal flap and remove bone to allow adequate access for the root to be elevated away from the antrum using a *lateral* approach.

Any root in the antrum requires removal as they always cause trouble and so the patient should be referred for sinus exploration and root retrieval. The remaining defect into the antrum from the socket also should be addressed (see section on oro–antral communication above).

Displacement of the tooth or a root into the tissues   is a rare but potentially serious complication. The tooth or part of it may be lost under a mucoperiosteal flap (Figure 5.6a, b), into the lingual pouch through the thin lingual cortex of bone in the lower third molar region, or into the infratemporal fossa around the back of the maxillary tuberosity from the upper third molar region. Ineffectual efforts at applying forceps to a tooth or elevating a root with inadequate access may cause such displacements, but occasionally this mishap occurs unpredictably even with sound technique. Any root or part of a tooth that is unaccounted for during extraction should be pursued by taking a further radiograph of the socket and, if possible, the surrounding area. The patient should then be referred for further investigation and management by an oral surgeon.

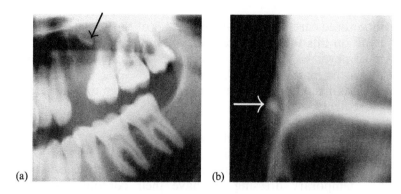

(a)   (b)

Figure 5.6. (a) A fractured portion of root displaced from the socket of the upper second premolar. (b) This cross-sectional scan view shows the root fragment to be under the buccal flap and not in the antral cavity.

If a tooth or root is lost from view during the course of an extraction, it may be in one of the following sites:

- Swallowed into the stomach or inhaled into the lung. If either of these is suspected the patient should be sent to hospital for abdominal and chest radiographs.
- Pushed into the antrum (see above for management).
- Displaced into a soft tissue space (as described above).
- Collected inadvertently by the suction apparatus (check the filter).
- Still in the socket.

Fracture or subluxation of an adjacent tooth during extraction should be avoidable using appropriate techniques with forceps and elevators (see Chapters 2 and 3) to ensure that these instruments cannot slip from their intended site of action to damage an adjacent tooth or one in the opposing jaw. In general, the rule is that no force should be applied to teeth other than the one being removed. Particular care must be taken when using an elevator between two teeth, and this should be avoided if the tooth for extraction is larger than its immediate neighbour, e.g. a lower first molar and second premolar. Some force will inevitably be transmitted via the interseptal bone to the adjacent tooth and this must be monitored carefully by placing a finger of the left (stabilizing) hand on this tooth to check for any movement. Direct force must never be applied to an adjacent tooth unless it is also due to be removed *at the same visit*.

Certain situations make inadvertent damage to other teeth more likely:

- Overhanging restorations in adjacent teeth. It would sometimes be impossible not to break such restorations, and ideally they should be removed and replaced with a temporary dressing, or have their contour corrected prior to the extraction.
- Bulbous full crown restorations on adjacent teeth. The utmost care is needed not to displace some of these crowns and the patient should be warned about this possibility pre-operatively.
- If the tooth for extraction is a bridge abutment, the bridge must either be removed completely, or sectioned to isolate the tooth to be extracted.
- Extractions under general anaesthesia pose possible dangers to the dentition from the injudicious use of mouth props, laryngoscopes, oral endotracheal tubes and airways used during recovery of the patient.

Collateral damage to surrounding soft tissues. A certain amount of disruption to the gingival tissues around an extracted tooth is to be expected. Some attached gingiva may need to be dissected free of small fragments of alveolar bone but such displaced tissues, like flaps of mucoperiosteum, can be replaced with sutures. However, the incidence of the following modes of soft tissue injury can be reduced with care and forethought:

- Gingival tissue lacerated by the forceps blades. Be sure to place the blades *inside* the gingival crevice and not trap the soft tissue against the tooth. This is a particular danger on the lingual aspect of lower teeth.
- Lower lip crushed against the lower teeth while extracting resistant upper molars. This is due to incorrect angulation of the forceps and is more likely

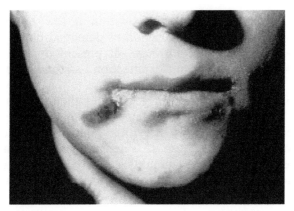

Figure 5.7. Burn to the lower lip caused by a handpiece that overheated.

to happen under general anaesthesia or when the patient's lower lip is also anaesthetized. Awareness of this problem is usually enough to prevent it.

- An elevator that slips off the intended point of application and stabs the tongue, floor of mouth or the palate. Elevators should always be held with the index finger down the shank of the handle towards the tip to act as a 'stop' in case the instrument slips (see Chapter 2 for the correct use of elevators).

Thermal injury to lips or cheeks may result from the continued use of a handpiece with worn bearings so that the instrument overheats (Figure 5.7). The surgeon cannot feel the rise in temperature until too late because surgical rubber gloves provide excellent thermal insulation. Awareness of the problem and regular maintenance of equipment will reduce the incidence of this unfortunate event. Instruments used too quickly after their removal from the autoclave may cause a similar problem.

Haemorrhage. Tooth extraction is a stringent test of haemostasis and excessive bleeding from the socket occurs not infrequently even in patients who have no pathological haemorrhagic tendency. The bleeding may be at the time of surgery – *primary haemorrhage*, within a few hours after surgery when the vasoconstriction of damaged blood vessels ceases – *reactionary haemorrhage*, or present up to 14 days post-operatively as a result of infection – *secondary haemorrhage*.

All patients should be asked whether they or any blood relative have a history of excessive bleeding and full details obtained about relevant previous incidents particularly following tooth extraction. If a haemorrhagic diathesis is suspected then the patient should be referred for investigation by a haematologist. Diseases causing excessive bleeding may involve abnormalities of:

- Blood clotting, e.g. haemophilia, or more commonly the acquired complication of anticoagulant therapy.
- Platelet deficiency (thrombocytopenia), either because of rapid destruction or failure of production of platelets.
- Blood vessels.

Precautions to minimize the risk of haemorrhage include careful handling of the tissues to avoid unnecessary trauma, placing a gauze pack over the socket for at least 10 minutes with the patient applying steady pressure by biting gently to encourage a blood clot to form in the socket, and then instructing the patient not to disturb the clot by avoiding vigorous mouth rinsing or chewing.

If haemorrhage becomes a problem at the time of extraction, it is essential to have good suction apparatus available so that clear vision of the operative field is maintained. Usually the source of the bleeding is the gingival tissue and more rarely the bone of the socket. Injecting further local anaesthetic solution containing a vasoconstrictor can help substantially to control soft tissue bleeding whilst a horizontal mattress suture is placed across the margins of the socket (Figure 5.8). A small pack of resorbable oxidized cellulose gauze (Surgicel – Ethicon) placed into the superficial part of the socket further stabilizes the forming blood clot at this site. Occasionally a single blood vessel is seen to be the bleeding point and this can then be tied off using a suture or coagulated with diathermy. When persistent oozing is coming from the cancellous bone, this can be stopped by smearing

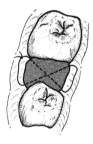

Figure 5.8. Diagram of a horizontal mattress suture placed diagonally across a tooth socket. This suture both helps to control haemorrhage from the soft tissue socket margins and stabilizes any pack within the socket.

bone wax into the relevant spaces in the bone marrow using the convex back of a Mitchell's trimmer. If all else fails then packing the socket with gauze soaked in Whitehead's varnish (compound iodoform paint) is a reliable solution to the problem but the pack must be removed 10 days later.

When patients return with post-operative haemorrhage it is often amidst a flurry of high anxiety and blood stained dribbling. Sitting the patient down quietly, cleaning away the blood clots that have formed in the mouth but evidently not in the socket, and giving reassurance while the patient bites on a pack placed accurately over the bleeding area will do much to remedy the situation. In some cases this may be enough to stop the haemorrhage. Normally it is helpful to inject local anaesthetic around the socket and then suture its margins with or without the placement of a pack. The medical history should be checked along with any drugs that are being taken, notably any anticoagulant such as warfarin, although aspirin and non-steroidal anti-inflammatory drugs have an anti-platelet action and may sometimes be the cause of significant haemorrhage. If it is thought that there could be a systemic rather than a local reason for the bleeding, it may be appropriate to refer the patient for further investigation. In the case of haemorrhage that is not controllable by the above measures, the patient should be sent directly to hospital for surgical management which in severe cases could entail admission and blood transfusion.

Dislocation of the temporomandibular joint   during forceps extraction is normally the result of failure to support the mandible while a difficult lower tooth is being loosened. The operator's left hand should ideally stabilize the jaw during

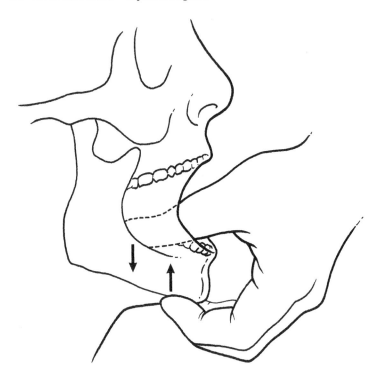

Figure 5.9. Method of reducing a dislocation of the mandible.

this manoeuvre, but the dental forceps provide considerable mechanical advantage, allowing larger displacing forces to be applied to the jaw than the left hand can resist. Additional support may be obtained by asking the patient to bite onto a mouth prop which then transfers some of the force to the maxillary teeth.

Some patients dislocate very easily and a history of previous episodes of dislocation should never be ignored. Dislocation is more likely to happen under general anaesthesia when the masticatory musculature is relaxed, particularly with the injudicious use of mouth gags to force the jaws apart.

It is important to recognize dislocation (by the induced class III jaw relationship and the inability to close the mouth into centric occlusion), and then correct it immediately. Reduction at this time is readily achieved with the operator positioned in front of the patient, thumbs wrapped in gauze and placed on the lower back teeth and fingers under the lower border of the mandible (Figure 5.9). By pushing down on the molar teeth and rotating the chin upwards, the condyles are moved downwards and backwards over the articular eminences of the temporal bone to regain position in the glenoid fossae. If there is delay in reducing the dislocation and resistance is encountered, the placement of local anaesthetic solution high in the buccal sulcus bilaterally adjacent to the upper third molar region (as if giving posterior superior dental blocks) will assist reduction by paralysing the lateral pterygoid muscles and overcoming the muscular spasm holding the condyles forwards. Under general anaesthesia, dislocations are normally easy to reduce once the problem is recognized, hence the value of always checking the occlusion at the end of any extraction procedure.

Fracture of the mandible is a rare event during dental extraction. It usually signifies that either there is some predisposing weakness of the jaw which then exhibits a pathological fracture when 'normal' forces are applied to a tooth, or that excessive force sufficient to break a 'normal' mandible has been used.

Examples of conditions predisposing to pathological fracture include:

- large cysts
- tumours (including bone metastases)
- impacted/buried teeth
- generalized osteoporosis
- Paget's disease
- osteogenesis imperfecta
- hyperparathyroidism.

When weakness of the jaw is suspected pre-operatively, the patient should be warned about the possibility of fracture, and the extraction planned to be conducted in an environment where this complication could be adequately managed by immediate reduction and fixation. Care and restraint must

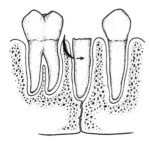

Figure 5.10. Excessive lateral force applied between the roots of teeth in the mandible may threaten jaw fracture.

always be exercised when applying force to extract any tooth; moreover there are certain operative manoeuvres that may threaten to fracture the mandible:

- Using an elevator that is too wide between two lower teeth thus forcing them apart mesio-distally (Figure 5.10).
- Using straight elevators as class 1 levers.
- Excessive bone removal, particularly if both buccal *and* lingual cortices are reduced.

If fracture of the mandible during the course of extraction is suspected, the procedure should be stopped, appropriate radiographs taken, and the patient referred immediately by telephone or fax for management by an oral surgeon. A full explanation should be given to the patient as well as a prescription for suitable antibiotics and analgesics.

Nerve damage. The following branches of the trigeminal nerve may be at risk during tooth extraction.

The *mental nerve* can be damaged by over-extension of relieving incisions in the depth of the buccal sulcus in the lower premolar region, or by bone removal encroaching on the mental foramen just below and between the premolar root apices. The affected area of sensory loss extends over the ipsilateral lower lip and chin.

The *inferior dental nerve*, of which the mental nerve is a branch, also supplies sensation to all the lower teeth and the buccal gingivae anterior to the mental foramen. The nerve runs close to the roots of the lower third molar which may impinge upon the inferior dental canal (including the nerve)

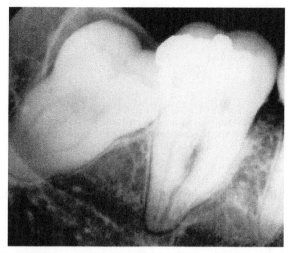

Figure 5.11. Lower third molar with a radiolucent band crossing its root indicating that the inferior dental canal (including the nerve) is grooving the root and is therefore at risk if this tooth is removed. The shadow of the canal is also deviated and narrowed where it crosses the root.

during extraction. Occasionally the tooth roots are curved around the canal or grooved by it so that movement of the root is highly likely to cause nerve damage. Pre-operative radiographic assessment of third molars is imperative to avoid inadvertent damage which results in temporary sensory disturbance in about 3% of cases, and permanent numbness of the lower lip in 0.5% of lower third molar extractions. There are three radiographic signs of close proximity of the nerve and root (Figure 5.11):

(1) *a radiolucent band* where the inferior dental canal crosses the root, indicating that the root is either grooved or penetrated, hence there is less dentine to attenuate the X-ray beam (Figure 5.12);

(2) *deviation of the canal*; and

(3) *narrowing of the canal.*

Some authorities also include the loss of the cortical outline of the canal – the 'tramlines'. This, however, is not a reliable sign.

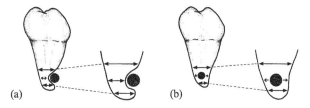

Figure 5.12. Diagrams to show the reduction of X-ray beam attenuation where the root dentine is thinned as the inferior dental canal either (a) grooves or (b) penetrates the root of a lower third molar.

In cases where there is an intimate relationship between root and nerve, the patient should be referred for specialist advice and treatment.

The *lingual nerve* also has a course close to the lower third molar as it passes the mandible in this region, often in contact with the lingual periosteum. Therefore this nerve is at risk of crush injury during periosteal elevation lingual to the lower third molar, or of direct trauma from burs and chisels used to remove bone. The incidence of permanent sensory loss in the tongue (which also includes the special sense of taste) following third molar removal is 0.5%, and temporary numbness is reported to be as high as 10% in some series.

Whenever the operative field of an extraction is likely to involve tissues close to these sensory nerves, the patient should be given appropriate pre-operative warnings about the possible dangers as well as the probable outcome.

Excessive pain, swelling and trismus.   Some degree of swelling and discomfort is to be expected after any surgical procedure; tooth extraction is no exception. Suitable analgesic medication prescribed for the patient *before* the expected onset of pain, combined with appropriate post-operative instructions and reassurance, is normally adequate management of these symptoms. Careful instrumentation and handling of the tissues during surgery minimizes post-operative oedema by avoiding unnecessary trauma, but other causes of swelling, such as haematoma formation or infection, cannot always be prevented.

Trismus is an inability to open the mouth to a normal gape,

and is commonly seen following extractions, particularly lower molars. Inflammation and oedema may spread from this region to affect the powerful jaw closing muscles, masseter and medial pterygoid, which are then painful when stretched. Severe and progressive trismus occasionally follows a few days after an inferior dental nerve block as the result of the development of a haematoma in the medial pterygoid muscle. The passage of the local anaesthetic needle through this muscle may unavoidably pierce a small blood vessel and cause some bleeding between the muscle fibres. Fibrosis of the haematoma may result in prolonged limitation of mouth opening unless active stretching exercises are employed. Trismus due to oedema normally resolves spontaneously with the inflammation but the patient can be made more comfortable meanwhile by the application of heat to the affected area.

Dry socket is characterized by the onset of acute pain and a foul odour a few days post extraction. There is lysis of the blood clot in the socket, exposing vital bone which is exquisitely tender to touch. The socket margins may have a greyish sloughing appearance but there is no suppuration. The healing of the socket is delayed by this inflammatory process and pain normally continues for at least 10–14 days. Although not strictly an infective lesion, bacteria, notably anaerobes, may play a part in the aetio-pathogenesis of dry socket, and the prophylactic use of antimicrobial drugs such as metronidazole and clindamycin have been shown to reduce its incidence. The overall incidence of dry socket is reported to be between 1 and 3% for all extractions other than lower third molars where it may be up to 10 times higher. There are a number of predisposing factors:

- Excessive over-enthusiastic mouth rinsing leading to loss of the blood clot from the socket.
- Fibrinolysis – tissue activators released from damaged bone convert plasminogen to plasmin causing break-down of the blood clot. Kinins are also activated, so producing the pain.
- Excessive use of local anaesthetic containing a vasocon-

strictor, which may preclude the formation of a satisfactory blood clot, especially if the solution is injected directly into the intra-ligamental space.
- Greater surgical disruption and therefore tissue damage.
- Higher incidence in the posterior mandible than other parts of the jaws. Rare in the maxilla.
- Dry socket is more prevalent in females.
- Smoking.

Once established, a dry socket can be managed to ameliorate the distressing symptoms but there will inevitably be protracted healing of the socket regardless of treatment provided. Gentle irrigation of the socket to remove debris and any loose bone particles should be carried out using warm saline and a sedative dressing on a small piece of ribbon gauze inserted into the opening of the wound. Various proprietary brands of 'dry socket pastes' are available based on formulations with eugenol, balsam of Peru and often containing a topical local anaesthetic. The patient may need to be seen several times and the dressing renewed every few days to maintain the pain relief. However, it must be appreciated that any pack placed into the wound is a foreign body that may further delay healing, and that all non-resorbable dressings require removal. Adequate analgesic medication will be required until the socket has granulated over the exposed bone; antibiotics, however, are not indicated in the treatment of an established dry socket.

Post-operative infections are normally caused by anaerobic (*Prevotella, Porphyromonas* spp.) or facultative anaerobic bacteria (Streptococci) that are commensal in the mouth. Spreading inflammation around the extraction site gives rise to symptoms of pain and swelling that tend to increase in severity in contrast to post-surgical swelling that is reducing after about 48 hours. Pyogenic infections may lead to large collections of pus in the tissue planes and these abscesses must be drained as a priority in the treatment of the infection. Abscesses that present as fluctuant swellings in the buccal sulcus can be drained readily with an incision made through the mucosa (Figure 5.13). Deeper tissue space abscesses may

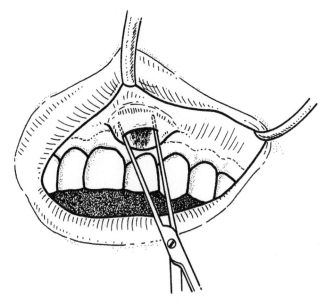

Figure 5.13. Drainage of an abscess pointing into the buccal sulcus.

require incision and drainage, often via an extra-oral approach under general anaesthesia in hospital. Antibiotic therapy is also indicated for any infection spreading locally, or where there is evidence of systemic involvement (pyrexia, malaise, loss of appetite). Tissue space abscesses from dento-facial infections can be very serious or even life-threatening, and any patient in whom such an infection undergoes rapid spread, or does not respond promptly to first-line treatment, should be referred for immediate management in hospital. This is vitally important if the swelling is involving the floor of the mouth and the oropharynx as further spread of oedema to the glottis may compromise the airway. These events can take place at frightening speed within the course of a few hours, and this condition, known as Ludwig's angina, has been the cause of some rare but tragic deaths in the United Kingdom even in the late 1990s.

Failure of the socket to heal after a period of more than 2–3 weeks is an uncommon complication that may indicate the

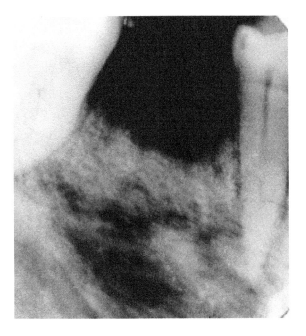

Figure 5.14. Radiographic appearance of chronic suppurative osteomyelitis following extraction of a lower first molar. Irregular patchy radiolucent areas surround more radiodense sequestra of dead and dying bone.

presence of an infected retained root or a piece of dead bone (sequestrum). More rarely, the socket may be found to be full of a malignant tumour, either from the maxillary antrum or a secondary metastasis within the bone of the jaws. Persisting infections of bone (osteomyelitis) and oro–antral fistulae may also be the cause of the problem. Any socket that does not heal normally should be investigated further; the cause may either be easily treatable, or may be the presenting feature of significant underlying disease.

Osteomyelitis is an established infection within bone tissue. Given that all tooth sockets are bony wounds open to the contaminated environment of the mouth, it is surprising that infections of the jaws are not seen more often following tooth extraction. The excellent blood supply of the facial bones as well as the immunological and anti-bacterial activity of saliva are largely responsible for this effect.

Intense penetrating bone pain, prolonged healing of the socket, anaesthesia of the lower lip and general malaise are the symptoms of osteomyelitis which, in the acute phase, may show signs of spreading infection and fever. If the infection becomes chronic the main features are suppuration, an indurated swelling, and patchy radiolucency seen on radiographs of the affected bone (Figure 5.14). Treatment of acute osteomyelitis requires a high dose of an appropriate antibiotic for an extended period, normally several weeks. In addition to this, chronic suppurative osteomyelitis demands surgical debridement of the affected area to remove any sequestra of dead bone.

Osteoradionecrosis is an extremely serious complication of radiotherapy to the jaws that can be triggered by tooth extraction. The effect of radiation on the tissues, especially bone, is to reduce dramatically their blood supply, and therefore to increase vulnerability to infection and failure of normal healing. All teeth in the anticipated radiation field that may require extraction should ideally be removed before the patient has radiotherapy treatment or within a few weeks of it (the ischaemic post-irradiation effects on bone are slowly progressive over a period of months). If the opportunity for this pre-emptive management has been missed and a patient who has had radiotherapy needs a dental extraction in an affected part of the jaws, then this should be undertaken in hospital by an oral surgeon.

Index